Advances in Dentures - Prosthetic Solutions, Materials and Technologies

Edited by Lavinia Cosmina Ardelean and Laura-Cristina Rusu

Published in London, United Kingdom

Advances in Dentures - Prosthetic Solutions, Materials and Technologies
http://dx.doi.org/10.5772/intechopen.111299
Edited by Lavinia Cosmina Ardelean and Laura-Cristina Rusu

Contributors
Alexandra Roi, Alisia Pricop, Anca Jivanescu, Andreea Codruţa Novac, Borislav Dusan Caplar, Ciprian Roi, Codruţa Victoria Ţigmeanu, Cosmin Sinescu, Cristiana Cuzic, Daniela Maria Pop, Emanuel Adrian Bratu, Emanuela Lidia Crăciunescu, Emna Boudabous, Ille Codruta, Ines Azouzi, Ioan Achim Borsanu, Laura-Cristina Rusu, Laura Rusu, Lavinia Cosmina Ardelean, Marius Octavian Pricop, Meda-Lavinia Negrutiu, Mihai Romînu, Mircea Riviş, Ovidiu Stefan Cuzic, Radu Marcel Negru, Ralph-Alexandru Erdelyi, Raul Rotar, Rim Kallala, Saied H. Mohamed, Sergiu Manuel Antonie, Yosra Gassara, Zohra Nouira

First published in London, United Kingdom, 2024 by IntechOpen
IntechOpen is the global imprint of INTECHOPEN LIMITED, registered in England and Wales, registration number: 11086078, 167-169 Great Portland Street, London, W1W 5PF, United Kingdom

British Library Cataloguing-in-Publication Data
A catalogue record for this book is available from the British Library

Additional hard and PDF copies can be obtained from orders@intechopen.com

Advances in Dentures - Prosthetic Solutions, Materials and Technologies
Edited by Lavinia Cosmina Ardelean and Laura-Cristina Rusu
p. cm.

This title is part of the Dentistry Book Series, Volume 17
Topic: Prosthodontics and Implant Dentistry
Series Editor: Sergio Alexandre Gehrke
Topic Editor: Wen Lin Chai
Associate Topic Editor: Ghee Seong Lim

Print ISBN 978-1-83768-235-5
Online ISBN 978-1-83768-236-2
eBook (PDF) ISBN 978-1-83768-237-9
ISSN 2631-6218

For EU product safety concerns:
IN TECH d.o.o., Prolaz Marije Krucifikse Kozulić 3, 51000 Rijeka, Croatia,
info@intechopen.com or visit our website at intechopen.com.

IntechOpen Book Series
Dentistry
Volume 17

Aims and Scope of the Series

This book series will offer a comprehensive overview of recent research trends as well as clinical applications within different specialties of dentistry. Topics will include overviews of the health of the oral cavity, from prevention and care to different treatments for the rehabilitation of problems that may affect the organs and/or tissues present. The different areas of dentistry will be explored, with the aim of disseminating knowledge and providing readers with new tools for the comprehensive treatment of their patients with greater safety and with current techniques. Ongoing issues, recent advances, and future diagnostic approaches and therapeutic strategies will also be discussed. This series of books will focus on various aspects of the properties and results obtained by the various treatments available, whether preventive or curative.

Meet the Series Editor

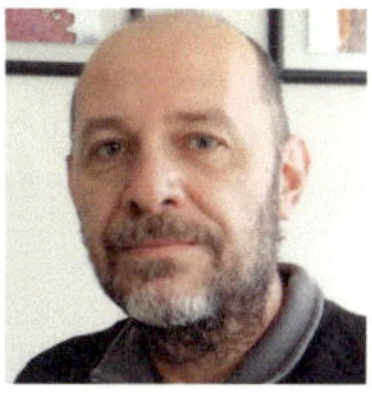

Dr. Sergio Alexandre Gehrke is a doctorate holder in two fields. The first is a Ph.D. in Cellular and Molecular Biology from the Pontificia Catholic University, Porto Alegre, Brazil, in 2010 and the other is an International Ph.D. in Bioengineering from the Universidad Miguel Hernandez, Elche/Alicante, Spain, obtained in 2020. In 2018, he completed a postdoctoral fellowship in Materials Engineering in the NUCLEMAT of the Pontificia Catholic University, Porto Alegre, Brazil. He is currently the Director of the Postgraduate Program in Implantology of the Bioface/UCAM/PgO (Montevideo, Uruguay), Director of the Cathedra of Biotechnology of the Catholic University of Murcia (Murcia, Spain), an Extraordinary Full Professor of the Catholic University of Murcia (Murcia, Spain) as well as the Director of the private center of research Biotecnos – Technology and Science (Montevideo, Uruguay). Applied biomaterials, cellular and molecular biology, and dental implants are among his research interests. He has published several original papers in renowned journals. In addition, he is also a Collaborating Professor in several Postgraduate programs at different universities all over the world.

Meet the Volume Editors

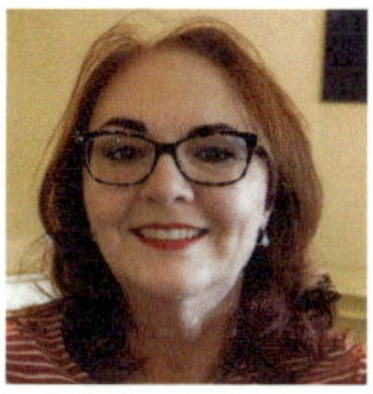

Professor Lavinia Cosmina Ardelean, DMD, Ph.D., is a professor and head of the Department of Technology of Materials and Devices in Dental Medicine, "Victor Babes" University of Medicine and Pharmacy, Timisoara, Romania. She has authored/co-authored 17 books, 14 book chapters, and more than 120 peer-reviewed papers. She is an editorial board member of numerous journals and a member of reviewer/topic boards of *Materials*; *Prosthesis*; *Metals*; *Coatings*; *Polymers*; and the *Journal of Functional Biomaterials*. She has guest-edited ten special issues in different journals and five books. She is currently involved in one ongoing book editing project. With more than 270 reviews to her credit to date, Dr. Ardelean was awarded two Top Peer Reviewer Awards in 2019. She currently holds two patents. Her research interests include most areas of dentistry, with a focus on dental materials/biomaterials, dental alloys, resins, ceramics/bioceramics, CAD/CAM milling, 3D printing/bioprinting in dentistry, welding, scanning, prosthodontics, and oral health care.

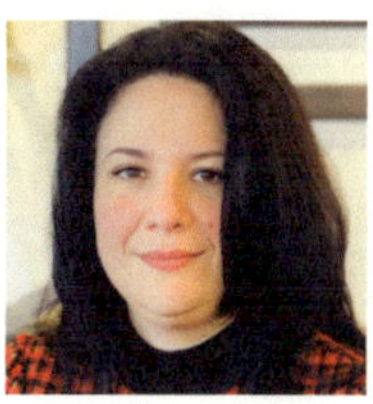

Professor Laura Cristina Rusu, DMD, Ph.D., is the mother of two lovely boys and a full-time professor and head of the Oral Pathology Department, Faculty of Dental Medicine, "Victor Babes" University of Medicine and Pharmacy, Timisoara, Romania. Her Ph.D. thesis was centered on allergens in dental materials. In 2017 she obtained a Dr. Habil and was confirmed as Ph.D. coordinator in dental medicine. She took part in 11 research projects, including FP7 COST Action MP 1005, and authored more than 140 peer-reviewed papers. She has published ten books and book chapters as author and co-author. She has guest-edited seven special issues in different journals, and edited or co-edited five books, plus one ongoing book editing project. She currently holds three patents. Dr. Rusu is an editorial board member for the *Journal of Science and Art* and *Medicine in Evolution*. She is also a topic editor for the journal *Materials*. Her main scientific interests are oral pathology and oral diagnosis in dental medicine, focusing on oral cancer.

Contents

Preface

Everyday activities such as talking and eating are usually taken for granted, but even these basic tasks become problematic if some or all of a person's teeth are missing. However, missing or damaged teeth are no longer the end of a beautiful smile. Modern dentures have advanced way beyond the removable ones our grandparents used to wear. Currently, a variety of high-tech and highly effective teeth replacement solutions are available, aiming to fully restore both function and esthetics.

There is a continuous and clear need for novel prosthetic solutions that support improved oral health and encourage patient compliance. Dental implants are more frequently and easily accepted as a common prosthetic solution due to the great progress made in this area of oral rehabilitation and the notable advantages of implant-supported dentures.

Dentures have highly benefited from advances in materials and technologies. Consequently, modern dentures provide a better fit and a more natural appearance than dentures from the past, resulting in fully functional prosthetic solutions. The metal infrastructure of both fixed and removable partial dentures have been replaced with better materials with improved physical properties and enhanced esthetics, such as zirconia, high-performance polymers, or injected resins. Flexible full and partial dentures allow for treating challenging cases, providing easy adaptation and better comfort.

The material properties directly dictate the manufacturing technology, however, novel prosthetic materials tend to allow multiple choices of processing techniques, their form being adapted accordingly to the specific requirements of the technological choice.

Digital manufacturing is, by far, the state of the art of current prosthetic technologies. While subtractive CAD/CAM technology is more frequently used for fixed dentures, additive technologies are better suited for removable ones. However, both allow manufacturing fixed and removable dentures as well. For sure, both CAD/CAM milling and 3D printing are here to stay and will continue to further grow in popularity, as less expensive alternatives come to the market.

In dentistry, 4D printing is demonstrating a beneficial impact, as the smart materials used have proven effective in the oral environment, which is characterized by continuously changing thermal and humidity conditions. Its application in prosthetics includes 4D-printed smart denture bases, with similar elasticity and thermal properties as the oral tissues. Additionally, 4D printing is being used to compensate for bone loss in cases of residual ridge resorption.

The choice of manufacturing technologies and materials, allowing complex prosthetic solutions and successful oral rehabilitation, is vital to delivering the best dentures to patients.

This book, consisting of eight chapters, focuses on complex and novel prosthetic solutions and materials designed for solving both functional and esthetic dental issues.

Lavinia Cosmina Ardelean
Department of Technology of Materials and Devices in Dental Medicine,
"Victor Babes" University of Medicine and Pharmacy Timisoara,
Timisoara, Romania

Laura-Cristina Rusu
Department of Oral Pathology,
"Victor Babes" University of Medicine and Pharmacy Timisoara,
Timisoara, Romania

Chapter 1

Indirect Restorative Polymeric Dental Materials

*Emanuela Lidia Crăciunescu, Mihai Romînu,
Meda-Lavinia Negruțiu, Cosmin Sinescu, Andreea Codruța Novac,
Borislav Dusan Caplar and Daniela Maria Pop*

Abstract

The current chapter, entitled "Indirect restorative polymeric dental materials," is dedicated to one class of dental materials with wide indications in dental medicine. The chapter is an overview of polymeric resin composites dedicated to indirect restauration currently used and latest avail resin composite and polymers in dentistry. This chapter includes chemical composition, indications, light-curing mechanism and physical and mechanical properties of indirect conventional and new polymeric materials. Important aspects about resin composites are related to clinical and physical properties such as light-curing, aesthetics, wear rates and biocompatibility. The accuracy and longevity of indirect composite restorations depend on choosing the right material according to clinical requirements, material's properties, and behaviour in the oral cavity and clinical indications. The chemical composition of resin composite, curing mechanism and advantages of these materials are presented in Introduction. The second section is dedicated to structure and composition of indirect polymers, indirect resin composites, first and second generation of indirect resin composites and their indications. Section 3 describes the structure and composition of high-performance hybrid polymers, hybrid ceramic and high-performance polymers, and poly ether ketone ketone dedicated to different processing technologies.

Keywords: composite resin, indirect composite restorations, reinforced composites, polymers, polymerization, physical properties, chemical composition, crowns, veneers, poly ether ketone ketone, 3D printing, plastering

1. Introduction

Resin composites, combined with best adhesive protocols, are elective dental materials for varied treatment plans and protocols offering a predictable, conservative and safe-working protocol. Composite resins are also designed for dental laboratory or for indirect composite restorations, being a multifunctional material without limitations in terms of esthetic or costs.

Resin composites were first introduced in 1958 along with the perfecting of a high-molecular-weight monomer, bisphenol A-glycidyl methacrylate (Bis-GMA).

Michael Buonocore noticed that some industries like automobile industry use phosphoric acid to chemically treat metal surfaces and obtain better adhesion of the primer to the metal. Three years before, in 1955, Buonocore observed that application of an inorganic acid can alter the enamel's surface and the bonding resin can be made. Buonocore applied this technique on enamel to enhance the adhesion of resin to enamel surface. He also experimented with acrylic resins but the occlusal stresses exerted over the indirect restorations in the oral cavity were too high. Rafael Bowen improved the system by developing a 25% by weight a polymerizing monomer and 75% by weight a vitreous filler-resin composite- and acid-etching technique, which became a protocol in restorative dental medicine [1–6].

First resin composites were self-curing resins obtained from a base and catalyst for which the polymerization was initiated chemically. The procedure was difficult but the material had superior esthetics in comparison with silicate cements, the elective dental material for direct restorations at that time. In the 1970s was introduced the light-curable resin composite which provided good physical properties, longer working time and better color stability. In the late 1970s were designed micro-fill resins with medium submicron particle size and the result was improvement of wear and finishing. In the following decades, the tendency in decrease in size of inorganic particles and increase in filler load continued and the result was the improvement of the physical properties of light-cure resin composites. Other factors that improve the physical properties are represented by free of voids resin composite and maximally polymerized organic matrix. These polymeric materials were continuously improved (physical and chemical properties) and are now validated as universal restorative dental materials [7].

Resin composites are also referred to as resin-based composites or filled resins and are defined as restorative dental materials made of synthetic resins and a matrix of organic monomer. Resin composite composition is formed by monomers Bis-GMA (bisphenol A-glycidyl methacrylate), TEGMA (triethylene glycol methyl ether methacrylate), UDMA (urethane dimethacrylate), HDDMA (1,6-hexanediol dimethacrylate), inorganic filler and a coupling agent, a silane which has the property to enhance the bond between the two components—monomer and filler. Other chemical constituents are added in different concentrations to tailor and adjust the mechanical and optical properties of resin composite [8].

These dental materials are classified after different considerations like handling characteristics, composition and size of filler particles, curing mechanism and direct or indirect indication of use. The direct composite resins are manipulated in the dental office, are placed directly in the oral cavity, modeled, light-cured by the dentist and are indicated for filling cavity preparation, diastema closure, minor reshaping of the teeth, built-ups and even partial crowns. Indirect resin composite restorations are designed in the dental laboratory and cemented in the oral cavity.

Conventional indirect resin composites have higher filler content and are cured for longer times and the deficiencies of the material can be better handled and controlled due to extra-oral design and curing methods. Indirect restorations made from indirect resin composites, after being designed by dental technician through different layering protocols, are cured at higher intensities and more accurately finished, polished and adapted to the natural or artificial abutment, abutment's limit preparation and proximal and antagonist teeth. The advantage of indirect resin composites designed for dental laboratory is that take benefit by curing under pressure, vacuum, inert gas, intense light, heat or a combination of these technologies, all generating a dense and completely restauration with no voids, less prone to marginal gaps and shrinkage.

In the same time, indirect restauration emphasizes excellent and functional morphology, and ideal proximal and occlusal contacts. The clinical recommendations for indirect composite restorations depend on the remaining tooth structure, cost and intra-oral relations of teeth and dental arched. Indirect resin composites are indicated for inlays, onlays, veneers, full or partial crowns on single teeth and even bridges [9].

One of the main issues of direct resin composites is light-curing shrinkage and degree of conversion but indirect resin composites can overcome these shortcomings because of modern materials and laboratory technological process. Indirect composites overcome some shortcomings of direct resin composite restorations because the material is manipulated out of the oral cavity. Clinical indications for indirect resin composite restorations always need to consider remaining tooth structure and possibility to properly isolate the abutment. Advances in chemistry, physics and field of adhesive biomaterials in the latest decade provide increased retention, reduced microleakage, improved marginal adaptation and good sealing for teeth or natural abutments and these successes of sciences completely changed the dentistry and clinical practice in dental offices. Modern polymeric restorative materials provide more conservatory dental treatments, which preserve tooth structure, and improve the longevity and esthetics.

Indirect resin composite restorations are also an esthetic alternative for intra-coronal posterior restorations such as inlays, onlays and overlays that reinforce the tooth structure and strengthen the cusps. The need for a conservative tooth reduction and in the same time good marginal fit and esthetics are recommending indirect resin composites as restorative dental materials. Additionally, clinical benefits of indirect composite resins include acceptable wear resistance and wear compatibility, ideal proximal contact esthetic and functional morphology [10]. The technological development from the last 20 years represented by digital impression, computer-aided design/computer-aided manufacturing (CAD-CAM) system and continuous improvements of dental ceramics, composite resins and adhesive systems are now sustainable for conservative restorative dentistry with excellent esthetics and mechanical properties of hybrid dental materials.

Until now, there has not been an ideal material for prosthodontic restorations. Currently, dental medicine has several classes of polymers used for the manufacture of fix partial restorations: light-curing composite resins, thermo-polymerizing resins, dual cure resins (light and chemically curing) and self-cure resins (chemical curing). Polymers represent a large series of synthetic resins, and composite materials are part of these classes. The very important stage in restorative dental treatments is the one in which the material is chosen as elective material depending on several factors: the extent of the dentition, the technical-material endowment, the manufacturing technique and time of use.

Composite resins in recent years have diversified a lot, so manufacturing prosthetic restoration is using these materials either through direct or indirect technique. Indirect composite materials processed through direct technique eliminate the laboratory phases though may face problems such as marginal and proximal adaptation.

Polycarbonate resins belong to the polymeric materials and are indirectly processed through plastering and injection. Because are thermal-plastic polymers, a special injection system is required. Glass fiber-reinforced resin composites are indirect materials that fulfil all the requirements for long-lasting FPP (fixed partial prostheses), with a maintenance period of time in the oral cavity between 2 and 5 years. Acetyl resins offer very good biocompatibility, this material is thermoplastic, and it is processed through thermo-injection and has some special mechanical characteristics.

All the physical properties of these materials have fulfil the clinical requirements and do not change different working conditions (chemical agents, humidity and isolation control in the oral cavity). Milling from polymeric blocks with CAD/CAM technology or plastering and injection of polymers are indirect techniques performed outside the oral cavity with new materials and technologies [11–14].

2. Structure and composition of conventional indirect resin composites

2.1 Polymers as indirect restorative materials

Polymers are one of the four materials that belong to composites and are commonly used as sealants, tooth restorative dental materials, cements, obturators for palatal clefts, impressions, provisional restorations and denture bases. The basic nature of polymers and the term polymer emphasize a molecule that is made up of many (poly) parts (mer). Mer ending shows the simplest repeating chemical structural unit that generates the polymer material. Polymer (methyl methacrylate) has a chemical structural units derived from methyl methacrylate. The molecules that form the polymers are called monomers (one part). These polymer molecules can be obtained from a mixture of two or more different monomers and are called copolymers (methyl methacrylate-ethyl methacrylate copolymer) and terpolymers when containing three different unis (methyl-, ethyl- and propyl methacrylate copolymer or terpolymer). In normal polymers, mer units are spaced and random orientated on the chain polymer. It is possible to obtain copolymers with arranged unit mer so that a larger number of another mers are connected and the polymer is called block polymer.

The mers of the polymers are linked through covalent bonds C−C and during the polymerization process, C=C double bonds are converting into C−C single bonds and the mer will be attached to one of the carbon atoms that belonged to C=C double bond.

The molecular weight of polymer molecule equals the molecular weight of mers, depending on preparation conditions. If the molecular weight of the polymer made from single monomer is higher, the degree of polymerization is higher. The polymers with low-, medium- or high-molecular weight molecules in a material or more precisely the molecular weight distribution have a pronounced impact on the physical properties of the polymer. For this reason, two poly (methyl methacrylate) specimen can have the same chemical composition but very different physical properties from a specimen with high-molecular-weight molecules. The variations in molecular weight distribution are obtained by altering the polymerization procedure. The spatial structure of the polymer molecules can be linear, branched and cross-linked and is important in defining the properties of the polymer. Polymers can be classified after setting mechanism, and these two mechanisms are thermoplastic in which the polymer can be softened by heat and solidified under cooling, and thermosetting; polymers that are solidified during fabrication cannot be re-softened through reheating. The variations in chemical composition, molecular weight, arrangements of mer unis, added fillers and initiators make polymer a versatile material with different physical properties [15]. In addition to being used as veneering materials, polymers are also used to make all-polymeric crowns or bridges. The most modern technologies are using CAD/CAM and the polymers used show remarkable physical and chemical properties, and can be inserted both as definitive restorations and as long-lasting provisional restoration. These restorations can be carried out either with the participation of the laboratory or only in the office. Currently, restorations based on polymethyl methacrylate (PMMA), composite materials and hybrid ceramics can be made using CAD/CAM technology. The PMMA blocks are made industrially and may contain inorganic fillers (which influence, among other things, the degree of opacity of the material) or prepolymerized organic particles. Some manufacturers also provide practitioners with pink blocks, intended for the bases of prostheses. PMMA indications in association with CAD/CAM technologies are as follows: single crowns, temporary occlusal veneers, provisional fixed prosthetic restorations (maximum 2 bridge bodies), for a maximum duration of 2 years and bases of prostheses. The basic structure of indirect composite resins does not differ from that of composites for direct techniques. Both are being represented by the organic phase, coupling agents and the inorganic phase (silicate macro- and micro-filling particles, made of glass ceramics or silica). Some products contain individual nano-filling particles or agglomerated in nanoclusters. With some exceptions related to the manufacturer, these materials are only suitable for single-identity restorations such as crowns, inlays, onlays and veneers. The resistance of industrially produced polymers for CAD/CAM technologies is higher compared to products with direct use, polymerized by a doctor or technician, which is also found in prosthetic restorations.

The modulus of elasticity of PMMA-based materials (2.7–3.2 GPa) is lower compared to composites (8–15 GPa) or hybrid ceramics (30 GPa), which gives the former a higher capacity cushioning of occlusal stresses and a lower susceptibility to fracture.

The resistance to spontaneous fracture is dependent on the Weibull modulus. The higher it is, the lower the fracture susceptibility of a material. CAD/CAM composites have a Weibul modulus (10–17) lower than hybrid ceramics.

The wear of CAD/CAM polymer materials is dependent on their composition. Thus, PMMA has the highest occlusal wear, followed by composites. Hybrid ceramic shows the least wear. Regarding the wear of antagonistic enamel, the highest rate is induced by hybrid ceramics, followed by composites and PMMA.

Water absorption is also dependent on the chemical composition of the material, being all the greater the higher the content of the organic phase. Thus, composites absorb more water than hybrid ceramics. Water absorption has a direct influence on the superficial dyschromia of CAD/CAM polymer materials. These differences are more common than in the case of vitreous ceramics.

2.2 Indirect resin composites

The first generation of indirect resin composites (IRCs) for inlays and onlays was introduced in the 1980s by Touati and Mφrmann. Direct resin composites were composed of organic resin matrix, inorganic filler, and coupling agent. The first-generation IRCs had an identical composition to that of the direct resin composite marketed by the same manufacturer and the material bore names similar to that of the direct resin composites.

The term resin composite generally refers to a reinforced polymer system used for restoring dental hard tissues. The proper scientific term is polymer matrix composite or for those composites with filler particles often used as direct-placed restorative composites or particulate-reinforced polymer matrix composite. Indirect resin composites are very similar to direct resin composite. Resin composites are composed of two phases, an organic resin matrix phase made from a mixture of multifunctional monomers and inorganic filler used to reinforce the matrix. Beyond these two phases, another two fundamental components are present in the chemical structure: the coupling agent (silane) that links the organic and inorganic phase and the different initiator accelerator systems. Additional chemical substances added in the chemical composition have influence over shade and other specific features of the materials. Organic resin matrix is consisted by monomers, the most common organic polymer matrix is a cross-linked matrix of dimethacrylate monomer and its double bonds at each end of the molecules undergo the addition of polymerization by free radical initiation with high-molecular weight and low contraction. These monomers provide optimal optical and mechanical properties. Because are viscous polymers, to be able to incorporate inorganic filler, need to be blended with low-molecular weight diluent monomer. The shrinkage of resin composites is limited by introducing monomers with epoxy functional groups at ends (oxirane). The conditions imposed to monomers from the resin composites are as follows: biocompatibility, physical properties similar with the dental hard tissues, chemical stability, chromatic stability and high reactivity. Conventional monomers, Bis-GMA, UDMA, TEGDMA and bisphenol A ethoxylate dimethacrylate (Bis-EMA) have been widely used because of their double bond polymerization mechanism that displayed satisfying mechanical properties for clinical practice. Bis-GMA was the first monomer for resin composites and is still in use because of low shrinkage but in the same time has a high viscosity and increased water sorption. TEGDMA monomer is attributed to cytotoxicity, low mechanical properties and high polymerization shrinkage, and in this regard, several dimethacrylate monomers including acetyloxypropylenea (acet-GDMA), bio-based ethoxylated isosorbide dimethacrylate (ISETMDA) and poly (propylene glycol) dimethacrylate (PPDGMA) were proposed to substitute the TEGDMA from resins because these monomers exhibit a close viscosity with TEGDMA, reduced volume shrinkage comparable mechanical properties and lower toxicity. The new monomers used for resin composites are as follows: methacrylate-based monomers, vinyl monomers, click chemistry monomers and ring-opening polymerization monomers. Methacrylate-based monomers are widely used for dental composites because of the double bonds of the polymerization mechanism. Highly cross-linked methacrylate-based monomer mixture displayed satisfying mechanical and aesthetical properties but their high viscosity imposed some limitation on conversion degree and incorporation of filler phase [16–19]. Research from the recent years introduces new multi-functional monomers; the use of vinyl, diallyl monomers instead of TEGDMA offers higher degree of conversion (DC), lower volume shrinkage (VS), optimal mechanical resistance and cytocompatibility [20, 21].

The appearance of click chemistry in 2001, thiol-X reaction has been introduced to formulas of dental resins and several kinetic advantages were provided by these monomer systems such as thiol-ene, thio-urethane oligomers and thiol-Michael's binary. The main characteristic is that the thiol-ene binary monomer system converts into polymer through a radical step-growth polymerization mechanism. Thiol-enes demonstrated several advantages when compared to methacrylate such as low amounts of unreacted functional groups, insignificant polymerization inhibition by oxygen and a uniform polymeric material. The ring-opening polymerization mechanisms, present at monomers such as spiro orthocarbonates (SOCs), vinylcyclopropanes epoxies and silorane, have remarkably attenuated the VS and shrinkage stress (SS-S) of dental materials. Polymerizing antibacterial monomers are introduced into resin matrix based on copolymerization among the resin monomers to overcome the short-lasting release of the antibacterial agents. The antibacterial effects occur through the contact of bacteria with the composite surface. The antibacterial fillers and following cationic groups such as quaternary ammonium, pyridinium and phosphonium are commonly found in the functional groups of polymerizing antibacterial monomers. Basic agents for polymerizing antibacterial monomers are quaternary ammonium dimethacrylate and quaternary ammonium polyethylenimine. Antibacterial filler particles can be part of inorganic matrix and are represented by silver nanoparticle, zinc oxide, titanium dioxide and bioactive glass. Antibacterial filler particles are water-insoluble and can release a small number of ions into the surrounding environment. Leachable agents are antibacterial soluble agents incorporated into the resin matrix and are released in the oral environment. The most common leachable agents are benzalkonium and chlorhexidine but their effect is for only few days [22–26].

Filler phase consists of various inorganic particles such as silica, silicate glass, quartz, alumina, zirconia, barium glass, strontium glass, hydroxyapatite, titania and ceramics and are being employed in resin matrix as reinforcing filler and tailor different mechanical and optical properties such as translucency and control of volume shrinkage. Beyond composition of filler, other characteristics such as size, shape, morphology, distribution of size and surface properties are modeling the behavior of IRC and the mechanical reinforcement is developed by a high content of inorganic filler (**Table 1**). Composite resins, studied with regard to the three filler contented, can be described as follow:

- low filler concentration—particles are in a non-aggregated form and only a small fraction of them form aggregated;
- intermediate filler concentration in which the particles are in close proximities to form a particle gel-like system and are called percolate particle network, known as percolating threshold;
- maximum possible filler concentration (specific to IRC) for which the network does not allow the incorporation of additional filler [27–30].

Size of filler particle and its distribution play an important role in the indirect resin composite performance. The early composites were macro-fills and contained spherical or irregular shaped particles with a diameter of 20–30 μm. The currently used resin composites are incorporating nano-size range and micro-size range inorganic particle size or a mixture of both and are named hybride, micro-hybride and nano-composites. The hybrid composites are blending two types of fillers: fine particles with a 2–4 μm in size and 5–15% micro-fine particles of 0.2 μm. The fine particles can be obtained

Composition	Size	Distribution	Interfacial properties and porosity	Shape and morphology	Content
Barium glass Hydroxyapatite Ceramics Zirconia Silica Alumina	Nano Micron	Narrow/ wide size Monomodal Multimodal	Surface silane modification Mesoporous structure	Spherical Irregular Fiber Nanotube	Non-aggregated Aggregated (percolation network)

Table 1.
Classification of filler phase-influencing factors on the properties of dental composite resins.

by grinding glasses such as silicate glass, strontium and borosilicate glass. Quartz or ceramic materials have irregular surface shape. Hybrids and micro-hybrids have good clinical wear resistance and mechanical properties and are suitable for stress-bearing applications but lose their surface polish with time and become rough.

Nanotechnology is produced by various physical and chemical methods, functional materials and structures at a range of 1 to 100 nanometers (nm). Materials with novel properties and functions can be obtained because of the very small particle size. There are two types of dental resin composites that are using the nano-filler particles: nano-fills contain nanometer filler particles with a range from 1 to 100 nm and nano-hybrids that contain large particles of 0.4 to 5 microns with added nanometer-sized particles and are considered hybrid composites not true nano-filled composites. Nano-filled composites combine the advantage of mechanical strength of micro-hybrid resins and service like micro-fill. The initial gloss of hybrid composites (micro-hybrid and nano-hybrid) is fading because of the difference in size of filler content. The nano-filled composited have similar matrix abrasion and the polish surface is kept on long term [16, 31].

Coupling agents from resin composites bond the organic resin matrix and inorganic filler during setting or polymerization with the use of compounds. These compounds are called coupling agents and are organic silicon compounds called silane coupling agents (is 3-methacryloxypropyltrimethoxysilane). Filler surfaces are treated with a coupling agent during the manufacturing process with following functions: to form an interfacial bridge that binds the filler to the resin matrix, enhance the mechanical properties; to manage stress distribution between polymer matrix and adjacent filler and to minimize water absorption.

Initiators and accelerator for polymerization are triggered by either light or chemical reaction. IRC requires specific conditions for curing such as oxygen-free environment, heat, pressure and vacuum. Heat curing is done at a temperature of 120–140°C and there is an increase in polymer chain mobility, which supports the cross-linking and stress relief, though prolonged heating can cause the degradation of the composite. Autoclaves, cast furnaces and special ovens can generate the heat source. An amount of unreacted monomer decreases during post-curing heating of the resin composite. In this technological process, two mechanisms are involved; firstly, due to heat treatment, the unreacted monomer bonds lead to an increased conversion itself and secondly, the heating is volatilizing the residual monomer. The combination of light-curing and heat increases wear resistance by 35% in contract with light-curing alone [32–34].

Nitrogen atmosphere is an isolating environment for resin composites toward oxygen, which inhibits the light-curing and thermal-curing. Once oxygen is entrapped in the resin from the surrounding air, it will weaken the restoration and increase wear and influence the translucency. The air removal makes the restoration more translucent and so, before curing the IRC is treated with nitrogen under pressure and the internal oxygen eliminated. Another method is the slow or soft curing, which allows greater level of polymerization; fast curing makes resin composite rigid and stiff. Electron beam irradiation at a usual radiation dosage of 200KGy improves the mechanical properties and positively influences the bond between la matrix and filler [35].

2.3 First generation of indirect resin composites

In 1980 was introduced the first generation of IRC and such examples are SR-Isosit Inlay system, Brilliant (Coltene, Switzerland), Visio-gem (ESPE, Germany), Dentocolo (Heraeus Kulzer GmbH &, Germany) and Concept (Ivoclar Vivadent,

USA). First generation of IRC had the same chemical composition to that of direct resin composite. Under light initiation, camphorquinone is decomposing and forms free radical and triggers the polymerization. The result is a highly cross-linked polymer but with 25–50% methacrylate groups non-polymerized monomer. For composite inlays, a secondary cure improves the degree of conversion but the only shrinkage that cannot be avoided is that of the luting cement. The effect of a secondary cure may vary among different material, post-cure though the post-light-heat treatment at 123°C increases the hardness, and wear resistance with 60–70%. The first generation has micro-filled inorganic phase and monomers with high shrinkage contraction for both phases and the developed properties lead to unsatisfactory results. The wear rates for heat-treated and non-heat treated resins are almost the same, around 60 μm in 3 years [30, 33].

The drawbacks of first generation were poor clinical performance; poor wear resistance; high incidence of bulk fracture and inadequate bond between organic matrix and inorganic filler, marginal gap and micro-leakage. At that time, resin composites were competing with ceramic and due to poor clinical results, the resin composites were abandoned when second generation of IRC was developed.

2.4 Second generation of indirect resin composites

The second generation of resin composites was mainly improved in structure, composition, polymerization technique and fiber reinforcement. The filler phase of the second generation is a micro-hybrid, 0.04–1 μm. Second generation of IRC had increased filler load twice that of organic matrix and as a consequence the mechanical properties, wear resistance and polymerization shrinkage significantly decrease. The resin was adequate for restoring the posterior teeth. Such composites are Artglass, belle Glass HP and Solidex (Schofu Dental GmbH, Germany.) having an intermediate filler loading with direct impact over esthetics and anterior teeth. Polymerization techniques for these resin composites are heat polymerization at 120–140°C and combination of heat with light increase wear resistance by 35%. Nitrogen atmosphere, electron beam irradiation and soft start or slow curing improve the quality of indirect restoration [31].

Artglass was launched in 1996 by Heraeus-Kulzer. The matrix composition is formed by Bis-GMA and TEGDMA (24–39 Wt%) UDMA-0.3 wt% pre-impregnated glass 60% for pontics and 45–50% for other materials. Artglass has a composition of 70 wt% filler of barium silicate glass of 0.7 μ and organic matrix of 30 wt% organic resin and four to six functional groups, which provides the more double-bond conversions. The resin composite can be light cured in a special unit using a xenon stroboscopic light to increases polymerization potential. The short excitation time followed by a longer period of non-exposure partially relaxes the already cured resin molecules and more of nonreactive double-bond carbon groups are made available for reaction. The indication is for inlay, onlays and crowns with metal substrate range from nickel-chromium to gold-based metals but in the same time can be used without metal substrate. Belleglass HP (Belle de St. Claire, US) introduced by Belle de St. Claire in 1996 has a chemical composition formed by silanated micro-hybrid fillers of 0.6 μ. This composite is available as base and surface composite for dentin and enamel with different compositions and five shades for enamel. The base has barium glass fillers as inorganic phase and surface material has borosilicate fillers that provide enhanced optical characteristics. For polymerization, Belleglass HP uses two different curing units that give the advantage of incremental build-up. The result is a natural tooth with the hard, translucent, enamel covering the more opaque and softer dentin, able to absorb the stresses. The base composite is light cure with conventional light-curing units to stabilize the restoration. The surface composite is heat cured in an oven at 140°C for 20 minutes. The atmosphere is oxygen free and under nitrogen gas pressure. The reduction in size of the filler improves the polishing and smoothness of the material. Newer composites have a filler diameter of 30 μ in the base composite, which will allow for further reduction in polymerization shrinkage. Other resin composite systems contain inorganic ceramic as micro-fillers. These materials have the advantages of both composite resins and porcelains without being confined by the inherent limitations of either ones. The filler particles are silanated for suitable adhesion to the organic matrix. The presence of these micrometric reinforcement particles acts as a "crack arrester," while the increase in particle concentration of the micro-fill particles provides improved clinical performance [32–36].

The design of fiber composite restorations is strongly related to the architecture of the restoration, which can be a single, frame or pontic, and the single and frame are glass-fiber-woven E fibers. Initial polymerization is for 1 minute with light-curing unit and final polymerization is made with light- and heat-curing units for 25 minutes. FiberKor (Jeneric/Pentron, US) contains glass fibers 60% in 100% bis-GMA matrix and the architecture is strips-like that contains unidirectional individual fibers. The initial polymerization is light curing for 1 minute with light-curing units and 15 minutes in alpha light. Other resin composites like Ribbond (Ribbond, US) are directly processed in dental office and need chair side impregnation. Connect (Kerr, Germany), Splint It (Jeneric/Pentron, US) and Everstick (Stick Tech Ltd., GC Japan) have braid or unidirectional fiber architecture and are pre-impregnated. The flexural strength and modulus of resin composites influence fiber volume, architecture and aging. The effective reinforcement is achieved when fibers are placed in the sides where tensile stresses are present. New hybrid composite resin restorative materials have replaced these materials [37].

2.5 Indication of indirect resin composites

There are differences between direct and indirect resin composite related to chemical composition, indications and manipulation. Dental practice is embracing new materials and processing technology, and now the growing demands for esthetics and predictable clinical results are achieved. Resin composites respond to many demands and can compensate many demerits associated with ceramic like high cost, risk of fracture, brittleness and wear of natural teeth. Literature reports many differences between direct and indirect resin composites according to laboratory, *in vitro* and clinical research and many studies have reported that the clinical efficacy of the indirect resin composites is superior to the direct ones. Other studies reported that the two materials are similar, and few reported that direct resin composites are superior to indirect ones. One of the main issues for resin composites along its history is polymerization shrinkage, which though was continuously improved. The studies demonstrated the polymerization shrinkage is less present for indirect composites because these require the application of curing with heat, light and pressure done outside oral cavity and even more the new composites are designed for CAD-CAM system or can be plasticized and injected. So, their physical properties are improved and the polymerization shrinkage is better controlled.

There are some important differences between direct and indirect resin composite restorations. Indirect resin composite restorations are relatively smaller in size as a result of extra-oral preparation and polymerization shrinkage and marginal fit is compensated by the luting cement. Indirect resin composites report higher resistance to occlusal wear than the direct composite with an estimated value of <1.5 μm/year. Indirect resin composites can be properly light activated under vacuum or pressure and as consequence exhibit greater conversion of monomers to polymers. The optimized conversion is found in improved hardness, polymerization shrinkage control, increased wear resistance, shade stability and biocompatibility. The morphology outcome, interproximal contacts and occlusal outcomes provide a good control and result. The filler contents are in higher quantities and this enhances the physical properties such as strength, hardness, marginal integrity and wear resistance. Regarding esthetics of indirect resin composite, this can be very easily individualized through a combination of shades and excellently polished though color and shade stability, according to the literature, may depend on the product, chemical degradation, stain retention, oxidized carbon double bonds, water sorption, dehydration, the presence of rough surface and poor bonding, increased filler to resin ration, decreased particle hardness and size. The cost of indirect composite restoration includes the laboratory work and additionally, there is a needed to increase tooth reduction to assure the insertion path of the restauration. Also, the luting layer of the resin cement may be subjected to shrinkage [16–18].

Indirect resin composites (IRC) are now having a wide indication in the restorative dentistry due to clinical performance and esthetics but with specific limitation that needs to be considered in the elaboration of the treatment plan. Indirect resin composites are used as esthetic laminating material for metallic crowns and replaced successfully the acrylic resin. The new trends in dental medicine try to completely remove the metallic cores, an achievable goal with the new resin composites, ceramics and laboratory technology.

Indirect prosthodontic restorations are designed in the dental laboratory based on the registration of dental arch and the natural or artificial abutments with a silicone impression dental material or with the digital scanning technology.

IRC restorations have indications for frontal and lateral teeth:

- inlays and onlays emphasize excellent morphology, marginal fit and contact areas but the reduction of the tooth needs to be more invasive for indirect restoration just to assure the insertion pathway of the restoration;

- laminate veneers are indicated for improving or masking tooth position, shape, size, diastema, color or congenital malformed teeth; enamel hypoplasia, fluorosis, abrasions, previously non-satisfactory esthetic direct restoration and diastemas;

- Jacket crowns;

- full coverage crowns, restauration based on implant-supported restorations; in cases where occlusal coverage is required as in patients suffering from periodontal conditions or bone and poor periodontal support requiring occlusal coverage;

- fiber-reinforced bridges/retainers.

The contraindication of IRC is teeth with heavy wear due to temporomandibular joint and occlusal disharmony, patients with parafunctional habits and the clinical situation in which the working cannot be properly isolated [18].

3. Structure and composition of high-performance polymer

3.1 Hybrid ceramics

Hybrid ceramics are materials designed for CAD/CAM technology, which combine the reduced fragility and increased fracture resistance of composites with the ceramic esthetics. The CAD/CAM technology led to the revolution of materials and their use in many dental applications and is using two categories of restorative dental materials: glass-ceramic/ceramic blocks, hybrid ceramics and resin-composite blocs with shades of natural shade (RCBs).

Conventional resins are cured with high-intensity light sources but RCBs are already pre-polymerized by the manufacturer being ready to be milled and have superior homogeneity, mechanical resistance and no polymerization shrinkage. CAD/CAM technology involves three steps: conventional or digital impression with an intra-oral scanner of the dental units, digital data processing with a program that delimits the dental preparation, restoring contacts and occlusion and creates in the same time the design of the restoration and milling from a block made from ceramic or polymeric material using a subtractive technique.

Hybrid ceramics are divided into two classes: first class—nano-ceramic resin blocks, industrially obtained through high temperature and pressure of composite resin coupled with ceramic filler (80% by weight) and second class represented by polymer-infiltrated-ceramic network (PICN) blocks with 86% by weight ceramic structure infiltrated by composite resin 14% by weight [38].

Resin composites and ceramics are the most common restorative dental materials combined in one material. The result is a hybrid indirect composite named PICN with indications for minimally invasive restoration like crowns, veneers, inlays and onlays and implant supported crowns. PICN is formed from sintered ceramic matrix, 86% in weight infiltrated with a polymer matrix (Bis-GMA, UDMA, UTMA, Bis-EMA or TEGDMA) 14% in weight [39]. This material is combining the ceramic and resin composites properties, though has superior properties toward resin composites and inferior to ceramics. The Young's modulus of resin composite is the same with the dentin's, while the ceramic particles assure the high esthetic. This hybrid materials are trying to compensate the polymerization shrinkage of the monomer matrix and increase the mechanical resistance through ceramic particles and is presented as a material for CAD/CAM milling systems.

The ceramic microstructure is depending on the sintering process, which significantly influences the translucency, chemical solubility, thermal expansion and optical appearance. For PICN there is a dominant ceramic network with leucite phase, zirconia as minor phase both interconnected with the polymer-based network. The microstructural characterization, in particular the size and shape of ceramic particles, plays an important role in the physical and mechanical behavior. Chipping of restoration made from PICN dental materials is due to ceramic's brittle character and CAD/CAM milling can induce micro-cracks, which can be repaired easily without the need for additional thermal cycles. PICN exhibits high bending resistance and can be designed at a reduced thickness. The first nano-ceramic material was Lava Ultimate (3 M Ultimate, 3 M Oral Care, US) and its compositions contains silica particles (20 nm) and zirconia (4–11 nm) up to 80% in weight. The force resistance reported by the manufacturer is about 200MPs and has indication for occlusal coverage, inlays and onlays but are not indicated for crowns [40]. Cerasmart (GC, Japan) is another nanoceramic material with silica filled and barium glass up to 71% by weight and a resistance force of 230 MPa. The material is indicated for single tooth restorations like crowns, cuspidal coating, onlays and inlays. Many materials are avail on the market with different filler and monomer combination and physical average properties around: 170–230 MPa bending resistance, 7.8 GPa elastic modulus and compression force resistance of about 680 MPa. The survival rate for 3-year clinical work is 97.4% for inlays and 95.6% for inlays. The characteristics of hybrid ceramics and their indications are presented in **Table 2** [41].

PICN as implant-supported crowns needs to have high biological properties considering the contact with marginal gingiva and even bone. The PICN must promote proliferation and spreading of human gingival fibroblasts and keratinocytes. The materials used for the abutments and prostheses have to promote cell adhesion that is a critical property for long-term stability of the implant's supportive tissues. PICN shows intermediate results between titanium and zirconia dental materials [42].

Paradigm MZ100 (3 M Oral Care, US) was the first resin composite marketed in 2000 as CAD/CAM blocks with different filler percentage: silica zirconia 0.6 μm up to 85% by weight with a bending strength of 157 MPa, similar to feldspathic ceramic.

Since then, other materials like starting from 2016, the Brilliant Crios (Coltene, Switzerland) developed different formulas for reinforced composites with amorphous silica particles <20 nm, glassy ceramic barium particles (<1.0 μm) embedded in cross-linked methacrylate matrix with a filling content of 70.7% by weight and 51.5% filling by volume. These are translated in bending resistance of 198 MPa and elastic modulus of 10.3 GPa. The elastic modulus is close to the dentin's and this imprints a favorable behavior regarding the concentration of stress in the restoration and minimization of fracture. The main indications are for onlays and overlays.

Tetric CAD (Ivoclar Vivadent, US) has a matrix composed of Bis-GMA, Bis-EMA, TEGDMA and UDMA nano-filled 70% with silicon dioxide and barium glass. The bending resistance is 273.8 MPa and elastic modulus has values of 10.2 GPa similar with dentine.

LuxaCam Composite (DMG, US) has a composite matrix in which silicate glass inorganic filler is embedded. The ration develops a flexural strength of 164 MPa and 10.1GPa close to the natural hard tissue. The material's physical properties are

Material characteristics	**Indirect resin composite**	**Hybrid ceramic**
Microstructure	Inorganic filler in resin matrix	Ceramic nanoparticles in resin matrix and ceramic network infiltrate of polymer
Optical properties	Medium	Good
Bonding properties	Excellent	Excellent
Advantages	Rapid milling, mechanical properties, possibility to be directly repaired	Rapid milling, mechanical properties, possibility to be directly repaired
Disadvantages	Optical properties	Optical properties
Indications for use	Veneers, inlays, onlays, overlays, crown, bridges with reduced number of elements	Veneers, inlays, onlays, overlays

Table 2.
Features and indication of hybrid ceramics.

recommending it for table tops, inlays, onlays, veneers, partial crowns, crowns and bridges up to three elements.

Gradio Blocks (Voco GmbH, Germany) is a highly filled (86%) resin composite based on nanoceramic technology dedicated to CAD/CAM milling. The value of flexural strength is 250–290 MPa and 15.5 GPa elastic modulus and a coefficient of thermal expansion similar to enamel and dentin [39–42].

3.2 High-performance PEEK polymers for CAD/CAM and heat and pressed technology

A recently new material is polyetheretherketone (PEEK), a high-performance polymer for definitive esthetic restoration, and is a colorless organic thermoplastic polymer from polyaryletherketone (PEAK) family. The polymer was first developed in 1978 and later introduced in engineering industry and medical field. PAEK (Polyaryletherketone) is a blend of high-quality thermoplastic and semi-crystalline resins. The members of this family differ according to the ratio of ether and ketone categories. The increased ratio, but also the sequence of the ketone groups, determines the rigidity of the polymer chain and increases the melting point.

PEEK polymers are obtained by step-growth polymerization by the dialkylation of bisphenolate salts. Regarding its advantages, PEEK has low water solubility (0.5%), and minimizes bio-corrosion avoiding in the same time the release of metal ions which can trigger cytotoxic phenomena, allergic reaction and inflammation of gingival margin. These features recommend PEEK for protecting abutment teeth and adjacent tissues. The aromatic chemical structure makes PEEK resistant to electron and gamma beam used for sterilization and this feature opens new applications and indications of the material in the surgical field. The main disadvantage is the poorly adhesive hydrophobic surface, and the surface contact angle is 0 at 65° that is not favorable in wide applications of fix prosthodontic but can provide a balanced stress distribution, and has excellent mechanical properties compared to metal alloys. The mechanical strength of PEEK can be enhanced by adding glass fibers (GFR-PEEK) or carbon fibers (CFR-PEEK) in its composition and become a reinforced material with even closer of flexural strength (170 MPa), Young modulus (12 and 18 GPa) values to human bone and dentin and better color stability.

PEEK is nonmutagenic and nontoxic to fibroblast and osteoblast, and exhibits lower susceptibility to biofilm development and no evidence was found about allergic responses induced by PEEK and in the same time shows favorable response to osteointegration and antibacterial properties. Though is a metal free material, PEEK has a gray color and esthetic properties can only be discussed in case of veneering with composite resins, which is difficult to achieve and various modification methods for improving the bonding are needed.

From its class of dental materials, PEEK has varied indications and applicability in dental medicine such as: long-term fixed dental prostheses, crown, fix partial dentures, post-and core, other fixed-dental-prostheses, orthodontics, oral implantology as dental implant abutments, abutment crown and abutment screw and as material for removable prostheses. Related to fixed dental prostheses, PEEK is a promising alternative to zirconia being less abrasive and properties more closer to natural dental tissues. Related to crowns, when PEEK is compared to zirconia, it shows more balanced distribution because of the elastic modulus and regarding wear, PEEK exhibits increased material loss, but superior flexural strength that protects the restoration from bulk fractures. Compared with PMMA, PEEK has the lowest marginal and internal gap values. Precise margins are essential for a successful restoration and PEEK has better marginal fit and internal adaptation than crowns with zirconia though both are clinically acceptable.

PEEK is an aromatic semi-crystalline linear thermoplastic polymer and was obtained by step-growing polymerization. PEEK consists of aromatic nucleus linked by ether and ketone groups and was developed from bisphenol salts and aromatic dihalides, and the typical reaction is the reaction between 4,4′-difluorobenzophenone with the disodium salt of hydroquinone. During melting, chemical properties do not undergo any change. The different resins of the PAEK family present similar characteristics such as: good dimensional stability at high temperature, resistance to bending and traction, mechanical and chemical resistance against wear. According to the manufacturer, these resins are compatible with reinforcing materials such as carbon and glass fibers. Its chemical structure provides material stability at temperatures exceeding 300°C, has a melting point of 343°C and is reinforced with glass and carbon fibers [43].

Depending on the possibility to modify PEEK at the nanometric scale and to overcome its limits, the material is classified as follows: PEKK polyetherketoneketone (PEKK), ceramic-reinforced PEEK (Bio-HPP), carbon fiber-reinforced PEEK (CFR-PEEK), PEEK reinforced with glass fiber (GFR-PEEK), PEEK reinforced with hydroxyapatite, nano-TiO_2/PEEK (n-TiO_2/PEEK) and nano-fluorapatite PEEK (n-FA/PEEK) [44].

The external structure of this material can be changed through different chemical processes, such as that of wet surfaces, which allows the formation of functionalized layers at this level. Thus, hydroxylated polymers (PEEK-OH) are obtained by reduction, carboxylated polymers (PEEK-NCO) by coupling a dissociated reagent to PEEK-OH, aminated polymers (PEEK-NH_2) obtained by hydrolysis of PEEK-NCO and aminocarboxylated polymers (PEEK-GABA and PEEK-Lysine) resulting from the coupling of amino acids to PEEK-NCO. Due to these chemical changes, larger amounts of covalent fibronectin are fixed to the structure of this material, and thus, it is allowed to apply higher pressures on the surface of restorations made of modified PEEK compared to those made of untreated PEEK [45].

Pekkton (PEKK) is considered a high-performance thermoplastic polymer, being easy to use and prepare, becoming the perfect alternative to ceramic and precious metal restorations. Being a member of the PAEK (polyaryletherketone) family, it was produced specifically for dental applications with a chemical composition that ensures the best qualities of all the materials in the same family.

According to the technological process, pressed PEEK has larger marginal gaps than milled CAD/CAM restorations. Related to properties and fix partial dentures, the material absorbs stress and protects the abutment, especially the connectors provide greater stress distribution than the other elements of the prostheses; however, the occlusal area supported the highest stress. As post-core material, fulfil the accurate matching to the root morphology and has similar Young's modulus to the dentin. PEEK requires composite veneering to be integrated into the class of esthetic dental materials. About 98% sulfuric acid for 30 seconds for printed PEEK and 120 seconds for milled PEEK were considered the ideal concentration and time of action for promoting surface modification of PEEK. Plasma treatment (He, Ar, O, H, N) is a quick, safe and effective conditioning method that shown excellent surface modification. Sandblasting with 110-μm particles for 15 s at 0.2 MPa generates better bonding strength vs. untreated PEEK. This method can be associated with plasma and acid condition. CO_2 laser treatments of PEEK did not exceed good results [46–48].

Compared to the rest of the materials resulting from this class of polymers, Pekkton (PEKK) describes both an amorphous and a crystalline phase and is the best choice from its family. In the primary phase, the macromolecules in the chemical composition are disorganized, in this form the polymer has specific elasticity. From the second phase, the macromolecules are presented in the form of linear carbon chains, knotted under the process of weak physical bonds. Thanks to its crystalline form, the material describes a very high persistence and rigidity. The difference between the amorphous and the crystalline phase appears at the moment of melting. At the moment of cooling, the amorphous material presents a low shrinkage compared to the crystalline form. High-performance polymers are clearly the way to go: flexibility of use, dimensional stability, hardness, tenacity and abrasion resistance are just a few of their attributes.

Compared to PEEK (poly ether ether ketone), PEKK (poly ether ketone ketone) both belonging to the same family of PEAK, exhibits an additional ketone group resulting in improved mechanical properties. The different organization of the polymer leads to different results regarding strength, stiffness, melting temperature and melting behavior. Compared to the rest of the materials resulting from the same family of polymers, PEKK has both an amorphous and a crystalline phase. From a chemical point of view, the crystalline composition is much more rigid and resistant. PEEK has only a crystalline phase.

Pekkton should not be seen as an ordinary material, but as a therapeutic solution. In order to increase the mechanical properties of the polymer, carbon and/or glass fiber can be added to its composition. Its remarkable qualities, the specific resistance of human bone tissue, as well as the biocompatibility and esthetic appearance of prosthetic works show that Pekkton is the most high-performance polymer today and is perfect for fixed prosthetic restorations. Both the flexibility and the typically relatively low weight represent clinically important characteristics when addressing implant-supported restorations.

Currently, several revolutionary materials have appeared, namely high-performance polymers that allow the production of very light and very resistant superstructures. Among these, we mention the two groups and they are PEEK AND PEKK (poly ether ether ketone and poly ether ketone ketone). The differences between the two materials are relevant:

- PEKK is at least 80% stronger than PEEK;
- PEKK has elasticity similar to that of natural dentin compared to PEEK which is much more elastic;
- PEKK is harder and easier to polish, while PEEK is softer and hard to polish;
- PEKK is recommended in definitive restorations, instead PEEK only for restorations of 180 days.

Compared to the rest of the materials resulting from this class of polymers, PEKK (poly ether ether ketone) describes both an amorphous and a crystalline phase. In the primary phase, the macromolecules in the chemical composition are disorganized, in this form the polymer has specific elasticity. From the second phase, the macromolecules are presented in the form of linear carbon chains, knotted under the process of weak physical bonds. Thanks to its crystalline form, the material describes a very high persistence and rigidity. The difference between the amorphous and the crystalline phase appears at the moment of melting. At the moment of cooling, the amorphous material presents a low contraction compared to the crystalline form. PEKK (Pekkton) should not be seen as an ordinary material, but as a therapeutic solution. In order to increase the mechanical properties of the polymer, carbon and/or glass fiber can be added to its composition. Its remarkable qualities, the specific resistance of human bone tissue, as well as the biocompatibility and esthetic appearance of prosthetic works show that PEEK is the most high-performance polymer and is perfect for fixed prosthetic restorations.

Thanks to its chemical and physical properties, PEKK is among the top high-performance polymers used in the dental field. The manufacturer (Cendres + Métaux) reports up to 80% higher compressive strength compared to PEEK. The identical characteristics of human bone allow better bio-mechanical integration than typical non-precious materials. While PEEK is the most characteristic member of the material family, it may not be the right choice for dental applications where esthetic considerations and long-term structural properties are of utmost importance. Products made from polyetherketoneketone (PEKK) are better option. The characteristic properties of polyaryl polymers are basic qualities of the material, qualities identical to all polymers that are part of the PAEK family. Thus, both PEKK and PEEK share surprising mechanical, chemical and physical qualities. High-performance polymers are clearly the way to go: flexibility of use, dimensional stability, hardness, tenacity and abrasion resistance are just a few of their attributes. Currently, several revolutionary materials have appeared, namely high-performance polymers that allow the production of very light and very resistant superstructures. Among these, we mention the two groups and they are PEEK and PEKK (poly ether ether ketone and poly ether ketone ketone). The differences between the two materials are relevant:

Due to its incomparable chemical, mechanical and physical properties, Pekkton offers a wide range of applications compared to other polymers (**Table 3**). As for mechanical properties, Pekkton represents the material that has the most similar

Advantages	Disadvantages
Very good weight-to-strength ratio	High cost
Increased comfort for patients thanks to the naturalness of the work, then the bite but also the sensation of the oral cavity	Laboratory technology
Fast processing;	
Elastic and resistant like natural bone, reduces occlusal stress;	
Resistance to abrasion and dental plaque;	
Compatible with all sterilization methods	
It has perfect dimensional stability	
Radiotransparent	
No thermal or electrical conductivity	
100% biocompatible, suitable for long-term restorations	
The density of the material is similar to cortical bone and dentine;	
Low specific gravity, less than 20 grams.	

Table 3.
Advantages and disadvantages of PEKK polymer in dental medicine.

biological characteristics to the human body. From these properties, we mention: density 1.4 g/cm3, solubility 0.2 μg/mm3, hardness 252 MPa, elasticity 5.1 Gpa, water absorption 8.7 μg/mm3, compressive strength: 246 MPa, bending strength 200 MPa, tensile strength 115 MPa, melting point 363°C. The advantages and disadvantages of PEKK (Pekkton) are described in **Table 3**.

The indication for Pekkton is as follows: bridges and crowns over dental implants having two intermediates retained with a screw type system, which can be plated with composite bond press crowns or prefabricated acrylic teeth, mobile restorations such as bars and telescopic crowns, transverse connectors, the base of the dental prosthesis, hybrid variants that have special attachments, crowns and bridges that have a maximum of one intermediary located between the pillar teeth; and unplated parts such as marginal collarette.

The contraindication for Pekkton is patients who are allergic to the material, crowns and bridges that do not have sufficient occlusal space—less than 1.3 mm, patients with bruxism and inadequate oral hygiene [49–51].

PEKK presents the same characteristics of the human bone, due to its chemical and physical properties. This is why it covers a high spectrum of indications.

4. Conclusions

Mixed metal polymeric crown (PMMC) were an alternative and the first attempt to improve the esthetic for fix prosthodontics that involved the metallic cores. For the esthetic component of the mix metal polymeric crowns, the metallic core is designed, which is veneered with a polymeric material. Both polymers without inorganic loading can be used, as well as composite materials, including photopolymerizable ones. To achieve the adhesion between the physiognomic veneer and the metallic component, macro-retentions such as pearl retentions, nets and loops need to be designed. Micro-retentions are made by sandblasting or chemically conditioning and increase the adhesion of the polymer to the metallic core. To improve the marginal closure, which, only in the case of the use of macro-retentions, can be deficient, chemical adhesion was also associated and obtained with the help of compounds that chemically condition the metal component. Among the chemical conditioning processes, systems based on 4-Meta, Silicoater and Silicoater MD or Rocatec gave remarkable results in terms of improving adhesion. Despite the progress made in the field of metal polymeric crowns, clinical studies show chromatic changes, superficial wear or even detachment of the physiognomic component. And for these reasons, it is recommended to avoid the use of polymers in areas subject to occlusal stress. The use of fixed metal-polymeric prosthetic restorations is recommended only as temporary long-term restorations or the plating of removable components in combined restorations (crowns associated with removable dentures) [15].

Modern veneering materials, regardless of their nature, based on poly-methyl-methacrylate (PMMA) or composite resins, obtain superior physiognomic effects, especially due to the possibilities of layering different types of masses (opaque layer for masking the metallic core, dentine, enamel and shades for individualization). The polymerization can take place at temperature and pressure or by introducing it into a photo-polymerization device [16].

Hybrid ceramic materials consist of a three-dimensional ceramic network (approximately 86% by weight) that is then infiltrated with a polymer based on UDMA (urethane dimethacrylate) and TEGDMA (triethyleneglycol dimethacrylate).

Due to this structure, the modulus of elasticity is superior to the other two categories of materials. Indications for hybrid ceramic materials are strictly limited to single restorations: crowns in the frontal and lateral areas, inlays, onlays and veneers.

In terms of translucency, PMMA has the highest value, followed by composites and hybrid ceramics. The translucency of the material is one of the factors that influence the choice of the restorative material in the case of dyschromic preparations.

Biocompatibility is positively influenced by the industrial process of block production. The well-controlled production conditions determine a denser structure and a lower proportion of residual monomer, by increasing the internal conversion rate, which minimizes the occurrence of allergic manifestations [17].

PEEK and PEKK belong to the PAEK family of high-performance polymers. PEEK has a crystalline phase, compared to the PEKK, which has both amorphous and a crystalline phase. Due to its physical and chemical properties, the latter is among the top high-performance polymers in the dental field.

Conflict of interest

The authors declare no conflict of interest.

Appendices and nomenclature

Bis-GMA	bisphenol A-glycidyl methacrylate
TEGMA	triethylene glycol methyl ether methacrylate
UDMA	urethane dimethacrylate
HDDMA	1,6-hexanediol dimethacrylate
CAD-CAM	computer-aided design/computer-aided manufacturing
FPP	fixed partial prostheses
IRCs	indirect resin composites
UDME	urethane dimethacrylate
TEGDMA	triethylene glycol dimethacrylate
Bis-EMA	bisphenol A ethoxylate dimethacrylate
acet-GDMA	acetyloxypropylenea
ISETMDA	ethoxylated isosorbide dimethacrylate
PPDGMA	poly (propylene glycol) dimethacrylate
VS	volume shrinkage
SOCs	spiro orthocarbonates
SS-S	shrinkage stress
PICN	polymer-infiltrated-ceramic network
UTMA	urethane tetramethacrylate
PEEK	polyetheretherketone
PEAK	polyaryletherketone
CFR-PEEK	Carbon fibre reinforced PEEK
PEKK	polyetherketoneketone
PMMA	poly-methyl-methacrylate
PAEK	polyaryletherketone

Author details

Emanuela Lidia Crăciunescu, Mihai Romînu, Meda-Lavinia Negruțiu*,
Cosmin Sinescu, Andreea Codruța Novac, Borislav Dusan Caplar
and Daniela Maria Pop
Faculty of Dental Medicine, Research Center in Dental Medicine Using Conventional and Alternative Technologies, "Victor Babeș" University of Medicine and Pharmacy Timișoara, Timișoara, Romania

*Address all correspondence to: negrutiu.meda@umft.ro

References

[1] Galan D, Lynch E. Principles of enamel etching. Journal of the Irish Dental Association. 1993;**39**(4):104-111

[2] Jackson RD, Morgan M. The new posterior resins and a simplified placement technique. Journal of the American Dental Association (1939). 2000;**131**(3):375-383. DOI: 10.14219/jada.archive.2000.0182

[3] Roberson TM, Heymann HO, Swift EJ Jr. Sturdevant's Art and Science of Operative Dentistry. 4th ed. St Louis, MO: Mosby; 2002. DOI: 10.1159/000330601

[4] Myshko D. Nanotechnology: It's a Small World. Washington, DC, USA: PharmaVOICE; 2004. pp. 34-39

[5] Davis N. A nanotechnology composite. The Compendium of Continuing Education in Dentistry. 2003;**24**(9):662 665-7, 669-70

[6] Terry DA, Leinfelder KF, Geller W, et al. Aesthetic & Restorative Dentistry. Houston, Texas, USA: Everest Publishing Media; 2009

[7] Murariu A, Dinu C, Agop FD, Stefanescu V, Topor G, Forna NC, et al. Composite resins - multifunctional restorative material and practical approaches in dental field. Materiale Plastice. 2020;**57**(2):276-284. DOI: 10.37358/MP.20.2.5373

[8] Craig RG, Welker D, Rothaut J, Krumbholz KG, Stefan KP, Dermann K, et al. Dental materials. In: Ullmann's Encyclopedia of Industrial Chemistry. Weinheim: Wiley-VCH; 2006. DOI: 10.1002/14356007.a08_251.pub2

[9] Türkmen C, Durkan M, Cimilli H, Öksüz M. Tensile bond strength of indirect composites luted with three new self-adhesive resin cements to dentin. Journal of Applied Oral Science. 2011;**19**(4):363-369. DOI: 10.1590/s1678-77572011005000011

[10] Fahl N Jr, Ritter AV. Composite veneers: The direct-indirect technique revisited. Journal of Esthetic and Restorative Dentistry. 2021;**33**(1):7-19. DOI: 10.1111/jerd.12696

[11] Porojan L, Porojan S, Topală F, Savencu C. Procedee computerizate aplicate în tehnologia protezelor dentare fixe. Timisoara: Editura Eurobit; 2015. p. 3

[12] Sinescu C, Gabor A, Zaharia C, Craciunescu EL, Pop DM, Canjau S, et al. Sisteme CAD-CAM utilizate în medicina dentară. Timisoara, Romania: Editura Eurobit; 2015

[13] Bacârea V, Ghiga DV, Pop RM. Principii metodologice în cercetarea medical. Tîrgu Mureş: Editura University Press; 2014

[14] Zanin, F.R.; da Fonseca Roberti Garcia L; Casemiro L.A.; de Carvalho Panzeri Pires-de-Souza, F. Effect of artificial accelerated aging on color stability and surface roughness of indirect composites. The European Journal of Prosthodontics and Restorative Dentistry. 2008;16(1):10-14.

[15] Sakaguchi RL, Ferracane JL, Powers JM. Craig's Restorative Dental Materials. Fourteenth ed. Missouri, USA: Elsevier; 2018. 340 p. DOI: 10.1016/C2015-0-01767-1

[16] Basudan TA, Alshareef SM, Alshehri AJ, Alkhalil HA, Alhowifi SD, Alhusain AM, et al. Differences of

direct and indirect resin composite and its effect on esthetic restoration. The International Journal of Community Medicine and Public Health. 2021;**8**(9):4622-4626. DOI: 10.18203/2394-6040.ijcmph20213575

[17] Douglas RD. Color stability of new-generation indirect resins for prosthodontic application. The Journal of Prosthetic Dentistry. 2000;**83**(2):166-170. DOI: 10.1016/s0022-3913(00)80008-6

[18] Agathian R, Manoharan PS, Rajkumar E. Indirect resin composite - a literature review. Journal of Advanced Clinical and Research Insights. 2021;**8**:13-18. DOI: 10.15713/ins.jcri.322

[19] Marxkors M, Meiners H, Geis-Gersthofer J. Taschenbuch der zahärztlichen Werkstoffkunde. Koln, Germany: Deutscher Zahnärzte Verlag; 2012

[20] Strub JR, Kern M, Türp JC, Witkowski S, Heydecke G, Wolfart S. Curriculum Prothetik: Band 2. Berlin, Germany: Quintessenz Verlag; 2019

[21] Rosentritt M, Ilie N, Lohbauer U. Werkstoffkunde in der Zahnmedizin. Stuttgart, Germany: Thieme; 2018. DOI: 10.1055/b-005-143308

[22] Podgorski M. Synthesis and characterization of acetyloxypropylene dimethacrylate as a new dental monomer. Dental Materials. 2011;**27**(8):748-754. DOI: 10.1016/j.dental.2011.11.013

[23] Podgorski M, Becka E, Claudino M, Flores A, Shah PK, Stansbury JW, et al. Esterfree thiol–ene dental restoratives—Part a: Resin development. Dental Materials. 2015;**31**(11):1255-1262. DOI: 10.1016/j.dental.2015.08.148

[24] Schoerpf S, Catel Y, Moszner N, Gorsche C, Liska R. Enhanced reduction of polymerization-induced shrinkage stress via combination of radical ring opening and addition fragmentation chain transfer. Polymer Chemistry. 2019;**10**(11):1357-1366. DOI: 10.1039/c8py01540f

[25] Ligon-Auer SC, Schwentenwein M, Gorsche C, Stampfl J, Liska R. Toughening of photo-curable polymer networks: A review. Polymer Chemistry. 2016;**7**(2):257-286. DOI: 10.1039/C5PY01631B

[26] Alansy A, Saeed T, Guo Y, Yang Y, Liu B, Fan Z. Antibacterial dental resin composites: A narrative review. Open Journal of Stomatology. 2022;**12**:147-165. DOI: 10.4236/ojst.2022.125015

[27] Wang X, Huyang G, Palagummi SV, Liu X, Skrtic D, Beauchamp C, et al. High performance dental resin composites with hydrolytically stable monomers. Dental Materials. 2018;**34**(2):228-237. DOI: 10.1016/j.dental.2017.10.007

[28] He J, Garoushi S, Sailynoja E, Vallittu PK, Lassila L. The effect of adding a new monomer "Phene" on the polymerization shrinkage reduction of a dental resin composite. Dental Materials. 2019;**35**(4):627-635. DOI: 10.1016/j.dental.2019.02.006

[29] Bacchi A, Yih JA, Platta J, Knight J, Pfeifer CS. Shrinkage/stress reduction and mechanical properties improvement in restorative composites formulated with thio-urethane oligomers. Journal of the Mechanical Behavior of Biomedical Materials. 2018;**78**:235-240. DOI: 101016/j.jmbbm.2017.11.011

[30] Bacchi A, Pfeifer CS. Rheological and mechanical properties and interfacial stress development of composite cements modified with thio-urethane oligomers.

Dental Materials. 2016;**32**(8):978-986. DOI: 10.1016/j.dental.2016.05.003

[31] Aminoroaya A, Neisiany RE, Khorasani SN, Panahi P, Das O, Madry H, et al. A review of dental composites: Challenges, chemistry aspects, filler influences, and future insights. Elsevier Composites Part B. 2021;**216**:108852. DOI: 10.1016/j.compositesb.2021.108852

[32] Leinfelder KF. New developments in resin restorative systems. Journal of the American Dental Association (1939). 1997;**128**:573-581. DOI: 10.14219/jada.archive.1997.0256

[33] Terry DA, Touati B. Clinical considerations for aesthetic laboratory fabricated inlays/onlay restoration a review. Practical Procedures & Aesthetic Dentistry. 2001;**13**:51-58

[34] Rominu M, Bratu D, Lakatos S. Materiale Dentare. In: Brumar E, editor. Notiuni teoretice si aplicatii clinice. Timisoara, Romania: Editura Brumar; 2003. ISBN 973-602-029-0

[35] Greer RW, Wilkes GL. Apparent reversal of physical aging by electron beam irradiation-further investigations. Polymer. 1998;**39**:4205-4210

[36] Janani K, Teja KV, Sandhya R, Alam MK, Al-Qaisi RK, Shrivastava D, et al. Monomer elution from three resin composites at two different time interval using high performance liquid chromatography-an In-vitro study. Polymers (Basel). 2021;**13**(24):4395. DOI: 10.3390/polym13244395

[37] Bagis YH, Rueggeberg FA. The effect of post-cure heating on residual, unreacted monomer in a commercial resin composite. Dental Materials. 2000;**16**:244-247. DOI: 10.1016/s0109-5641(00)00006-3

[38] Marchesi G, Camurri Piloni A, Nicolin V, Turco G, Di Lenarda R. Chairside CAD/CAM materials: Current trends of clinical uses. Biology. 2021;**10**:1170. DOI: 10.3390/biology10111170

[39] Facenda JC, Borba M, Corazza PH. A literature review on the new polymer-infiltrated ceramic-network material (PICN). Journal of Esthetic and Restorative Dentistry. 2018;**30**(4):281-286. DOI: 10.1111/jerd.12370

[40] Fasbinder DJ, Neiva GF, Heys D, Heys R. Clinical evaluation of chairside computer assisted design/computer assisted machining nano-ceramic restorations: Five-year status. Journal of Esthetic and Restorative Dentistry. 2020;**32**(2):193-203. DOI: 10.1111/jerd.12516

[41] Spitznagel FA, Scholz KJ, Strub JR, Vach K, Gierthmuehlen PC. Polymer-infiltrated ceramic CAD/CAM inlays and partial coverage restorations: 3-year results of a prospective clinical study over 5 years. Clinical Oral Investigations. 2018;**22**(5):1973-1983. DOI: 10.1007/s00784-017-2293-x

[42] Grenade C, De Pauw-Gillet MC, Gailly P, Vanheusden A, Mainjot A. Biocompatibility of polymer-infiltrated-ceramic-network (PICN) materials with human gingival fibroblasts (HGFs). Dental Materials. 2016;**32**(9):1152-1164. DOI: 10.1016/j.dental.2016.06.020

[43] Qin L, Yao S, Zhao J, Zhou C, Oates TW, Weir MD, et al. Review on development and dental applications of Polyetheretherketone-based biomaterials and restorations. Materials (Basel). 2021;**14**(2):408. DOI: 10.3390/ma14020408

[44] Sharma S, Bhasin A, Mantri S, Khatri M. Polyether-ether-ketone

(PEEK) and its application in prosthodontics. South Asian Research Journal of Oral and Dental Sciences. 2021;**3**:60-64. DOI: 10.36346/sarjods.2021.v03i03.005

[45] Kumar UK, Murgod S. Strategies and modification of polyetheretherketone for prosthodontic driven implants. International Journal of Oral Health Sciences. 2020;**10**:68-73. DOI: 10.4103/ijohs.ijohs_4_20

[46] Blanch-Martínez N, Arias-Herrera S, Martínez-González A. Behavior of polyether-ether-ketone (PEEK) in prostheses on dental implants. A review. Journal of Clinical and Experimental Dentistry. 2021;**13**(5):e520-e526. DOI: 10.4317/jced.58102

[47] Wang B, Huang M, Dang P, Xie J, Zhang X, Yan X. PEEK in fixed dental prostheses: Application and adhesion improvement. Polymers. 2022;**14**(12):2323. DOI: 10.3390/polym14122323

[48] Attia MA, Shokry TE, Abdel-Aziz M. Effect of different surface treatments on the bond strength of milled polyetheretherketone posts. The Journal of Prosthetic Dentistry. 2022;**127**(6):866-874. DOI: 10.1016/j.prosdent.2020.08.033

[49] www. Pekkton® ivory - high performance polymer for definitive aesthetic restorations on implants Pekkton® Brochure/Catalog 01/05/2015. Available from: https://issuu.com/cmmedtech/docs/cm_pekkton_broch_a4_1016.03.01.01_e [Accessed: June 6, 2023]

[50] Alsadon O. Evaluating Poly Ether KetoneKetone (PEKK) Polymer Used for Fabricating Fixed Prosthodontics [thesis]. England: University of Sheffield; 2017

[51] Papathanasiou I, Kamposiora P, Papavasiliou G, Ferrari M. The use of PEEK in digital prosthodontics: A narrative review. BMC Oral Health. 2020;**20**(1):217. DOI: 10.1186/s12903-020-01202-7

Chapter 2

Chairside CAD/CAM Restorations

Anca Jivanescu, Ille Codruta and Raul Rotar

Abstract

Dentistry has experienced dramatic transformations in the last 10 years once digital technologies have revolutionized the entire operational flow. From simple crowns and inlays, almost the entire range of fixed and removable prosthetic restorations on natural teeth or implants can now be made using CAD/CAM technology. The evolution of these systems has led to the need for a change in the mentality. Moving from analog to digital for these technologies involves equipment costs, software, and training time. For a dentist, the first step in CAD/CAM technology is to purchase an intraoral scanner and move to the digital impression. Then it will transmit the information (the. STL file) to a laboratory that will take over the design and milling task. However, if he wants to invest more, he will be able to make the final restoration with *chairside* CAD/CAM systems, without involving the dental technician.

Keywords: intraoral scanning, digital impression, digital workflow, cad cam materials, biocompatibility

1. Introduction

Digital dentistry is greatly benefited by the present digital revolution, which is bringing new materials, techniques, and treatment ideas. The dentistry profession is undergoing a considerable shift due to the advancement of CAD/CAM (computer-aided design/computer-aided manufacture) technologies and the advent of novel esthetic materials. The emergence of technology has significantly altered operational procedures and workflow [1].

Through the release of intelligent materials on the market that are intended to improve oral health care and, in turn, quality of life, dentistry has improved and will continue to advance [2].

It is now inevitable to switch from traditional treatment methods—which are laborious and prone to errors—to computerized ones. A significant impact of digital technologies has been felt in most dental specialties. The most noticeable advancements in the digital operational process have been in dental prostheses, which focus on the use of CAD/CAM systems and digital impression techniques [3].

In modern times, dental offices are using intraoral scanners more and more frequently. The principal factors contributing to this achievement are the decreased working hours for the physician, enhanced patient comfort, instantaneous viewing of treatment quality, and the ability to make adjustments without having to redo every stage of the process [4, 5].

A successful outcome depends on choosing the right material for each unique situation, which necessitates understanding each material's characteristics. The objective of the upcoming chapter is to investigate the benefits of novel methods and materials in order to gather data for an acceptable therapeutic outcome from an esthetically pleasing and long-lasting perspective.

2. In office digital impression – intraoral scanning

The impact of intraoral scanners (IOS) in dental offices has advanced to the point where it is impossible to ignore it. These devices have advantages over traditional methods of capturing intraoral structures, including reduced clinical time, improved patient comfort, the possibility to evaluate preparations during surgery, prevention of cross infections and impression distortion, and the ability to store digital models indefinitely [6]. IOSs have a variety of uses when paired with CAD/CAM (Computer-Aided Design/Computer-Aided Manufacturing) software, including single-tooth prosthetic restorations [7], fixed partial dentures [8], and dental implants.

2.1 Factors that can affect the precision of the digital impression

There are still several factors that, through their direct or indirect effects on the scanner and the substrate, cause differences between the digital model and reality, even though IOSs have made significant strides in recording the surface details of the object of interest. Ambient light, the distance between the scanning tip and the object's surface, the scanning procedure, the surface humidity, and the material of the scanned surface are the most commonly aspects that contribute to the digital impression distortion [9].

2.2 Ambient light

Most IOSs use a laser to record a surface's features, allowing a photo sensor to record the reflection's projection onto the surface. Thus, the position of each point of light projection is determined using a variety of techniques (triangulation, confocal microscopy, etc.). Although scanners have optical filters built in, the photo sensor records not only the light from the laser but also nearby light that has the same wavelength as the wave released by the scanner, which makes it a possible source of inaccuracies. High-intensity light sources have the potential to completely impact the surface, causing all the points in the scanned area to become saturated with artifacts.

When determining the position of the 3D object's points, different light sources produce varying results; the effect is particularly pronounced when using incandescent light sources. High light levels (2500 lux, comparable to the dental unit's illumination) can lengthen scanning times and increase the amount of information that can be recorded [10].

It was found that the ambient light had less of an impact when scanning a dark surface since light radiation was being absorbed. Additionally, it has been noted that gray structures, on which light variations have little impact on scan quality, get the greatest results [11].

A previous study performed in the Department of Prosthodontics from the University of Medicine and Pharmacy 'Victor Babeș' from Timișoara aimed to investigate the influence of ambient light on the accuracy of digital impressions.

The purpose of this study was to assess the impact of various settings of ambient light intensity inside a dental office on the accuracy (trueness and precision) of an intraoral scanner. A resin molar underwent a full crown preparation before being scanned with a high-resolution extraoral scanner to create a reference model. The workspace's six most therapeutically appropriate lighting settings were selected, and the preparation was scanned using an intraoral scanner (PlanScan, Planmeca). In accordance with the six light intensity settings, six groups were made: group 1 = 400 lux, group 2 = 1000 lux, group 3 = 3300 lux, group 4 = 3800 lux, group 5 = 10,000 lux, and group 6 = 11,000 lux. Despite some variations in the trueness and precision data collected under the various light intensities, these differences were not clinically significant enough to draw the conclusion that the ambient light had a significant impact on the accuracy of the intraoral scanning. Therefore, it is impossible to provide a preferred ambient light setting for the scanning process in a dental office. Overall, in the various lighting conditions that were simulated in this test, it was unable to attribute any statistical significance to the accuracy of the intraoral scanner that was used. From the clinical point of view, dentists consider it reassuring that ambient light conditions have little influence on the scanning accuracy because it means that there is a lower potential for external error when considering using digital impressions [7].

2.3 Object translucency

Translucency is another property of the substrate that might affect how accurate a digital impression is. This means that some wavelengths that encounter a translucent surface are either reflected or scattered by the object's structure.

Unlike waves that are reflected straight from the surface, interferences are caused by light that is scattered in the substrate and is reflected at various locations and angles. This results in a direct reflection pollution that the scanner records, decreasing the accuracy [11–13].

This distortion of the digital impression occurs even in the case of scanners that use the principle of confocal microscopy, which theoretically counteracts the effects of translucency by detecting point-by-point the shape of an object [14, 15].

2.4 Scanning pattern and scanning distance

The operator's chosen scanning pattern is another element that affects the accuracy of the IOS. Although manufacturers provide broad instructions on how to position the scan tip, these are frequently challenging to adhere to, particularly in clinical settings when a full arch scan is necessary. Consequently, a number of scanning patterns can be found: (A) scanning on half-arch starting from the occlusal surface from the central incisor, then the transition on vestibular and finally on the palatal one, (B) scanning on half-arch starting from the occlusal surface from the lateral incisor, (C) scanning of sextants with the same pattern, and (D) sequential scanning in which each tooth is completely scanned, the scanner having a "S" movement (**Figure 1**).

Most findings suggest that the scanning method plays a significant effect in scanning accuracy despite other research showing that the scanning pattern does not affect the quality of the digital impression when using current scanners [16–19].

The scanning distance is another factor that might lead to errors. It is crucial to know if specific scanning distances produce more accurate findings than others because it can be challenging for an operator to keep a constant space between the scanning tip and the recorded soft tissues or teeth during the scanning procedure.

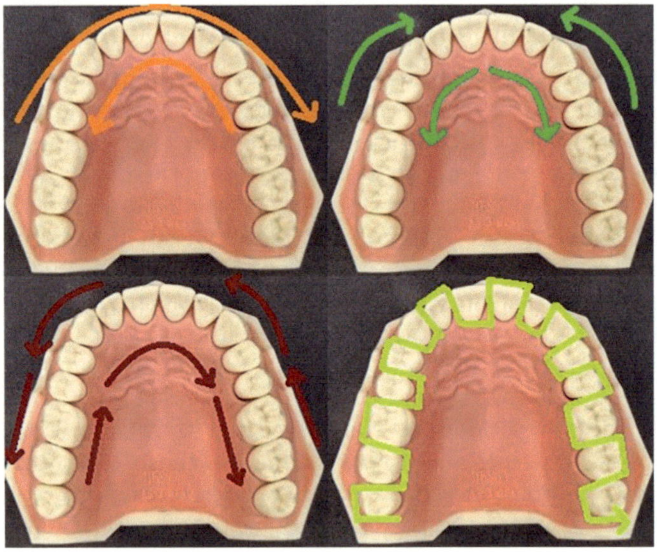

Figure 1.
Intraoral scanning patterns.

The objective of this study performed in the Department of Prosthodontics from the University of Medicine and Pharmacy 'Victor Babeș' Timișoara was to evaluate the differences in accuracy between digital impressions in the scenario of different scanning distances [20]. A single operator conducted twenty consecutive scans at five specified distances: 5, 10, 15, 20, and 23 mm. A previous study made use of the i700 IOS. The second molar and premolar's occlusal surfaces were recorded for the mesh alignment, but only the preparation's occlusal surface was scanned. The overall scanning time was 20 seconds, and the scanning path was the same for all distances. The typodont was moved in the following manner: Beginning at the first molar's occlusal surface, moving on to the second molar's occlusal surface, the second premolar, and finally returning to the original starting location. The typodont always moved in a straight line while resting its feet on a flat surface. The following conclusion can be derived from the study's findings:

- The accuracy of a digital impression can be affected by the distance between the tip of the IOS and the surface being captured.
- The accuracy of the digital model is decreased by close scanning distances (5 mm) or scanning distances more than 15 mm.
- The best accuracy was shown at a distance of 10 mm between the scanning tip and the prepared area [21].

2.5 Surface geometry

The geometry and type of the preparation in the case of fixed dental prostheses (FDP) is another element that may lower the accuracy of a digital impression. Dental preparations frequently deviate from the ideal occlusal convergence of the abutment parameters, resulting in areas with excessive convergences, parallel surfaces, or divergences toward the apical (negative angles). Guth et al. believe that a convergence of 6–15^0 is suitable for the majority of FPDs, although over 86% of the preparations under investigation had occlusal convergences of above 25° [21]. There is general agreement that scanners cannot catch these areas with negative angulation due to the limited access space for the scanning tip (in the interproximal areas), which results in lost data and decreased accuracy [22, 23]. Additionally, it has been shown that the accuracy of the digital impression reduces as the angle of occlusal convergence tends toward 0^0. This phenomenon is explained by the fact that the light wave occasionally cannot reach the base of the preparation [21].

2.6 Intraoral fluids on the scanned area

Another element that affects the accuracy of digital impressions is the presence of fluids on the preparation's surface. Even with sufficient isolation, maintaining an ideal layer of antireflective powder in scanners that use optical powder has shown to be quite challenging in situations when there are intraoral fluids present. The presence of saliva also affects IS (intraoral scanning) without powder because it alters the preparation's shape and surface properties, which, in turn, affects the reflection indexes. As a result, the scanner captures an image that is warped, which will negatively affect how well the fixed prosthetic restoration will fit. At the margin of the preparation, in addition to saliva, bleeding is also possible, which further impairs the intraoral scan. The blood's dark color causes it to absorb the scanner's radiation, which results in a lack of information at that level [24, 25].

2.7 Rescanning of the interest area

While it is often simpler to perform *in vitro* scanning by adhering to the suggested scanning protocol, *in vivo* scanning may be complicated by intraoral structures, such as the buccal mucosa and the tongue. The newest scanners offer rapid surface identification and data collection, although sometimes only one scan of a given area is necessary because the light emitted from the IOS cannot reach all of a tooth's surfaces, especially the interproximal portions [22]. These mesh holes may also be purposely created by the operator, for example, when the abutments are modified after the first scan, or when is necessary to cut off portions of the scan when overlapping of undesired oral tissues are present. The effects of digital cutting, rescanning, and overlaying of scanned surfaces on the accuracy of a digital impression have been studied in certain experiments [26, 27]; however, the outcomes can vary. Another study conducted in the Department of Prosthodontics aimed to determine which scanning method produced the most precise digital impression of a single-tooth preparation, whether data was obtained from a single continuously scan, a rescan to gather more information, or the omission of an area of interest subsequent to a rescan (**Figure 2**).

The following conclusion can be drawn from the study's findings:

The "SINGLESCAN" group provided the best trueness and the "RESCAN" group provided the best precision in the statistical analysis of the trueness and precision of the IOS scans obtained with the three distinct scanning techniques.

No specific scanning methodology could be suggested among the three tested methods as offering the best overall accuracy.

The investigated *in vivo* and *in vitro* instances showed no significant clinical differences in terms of trueness and precision. While the precision results varied slightly

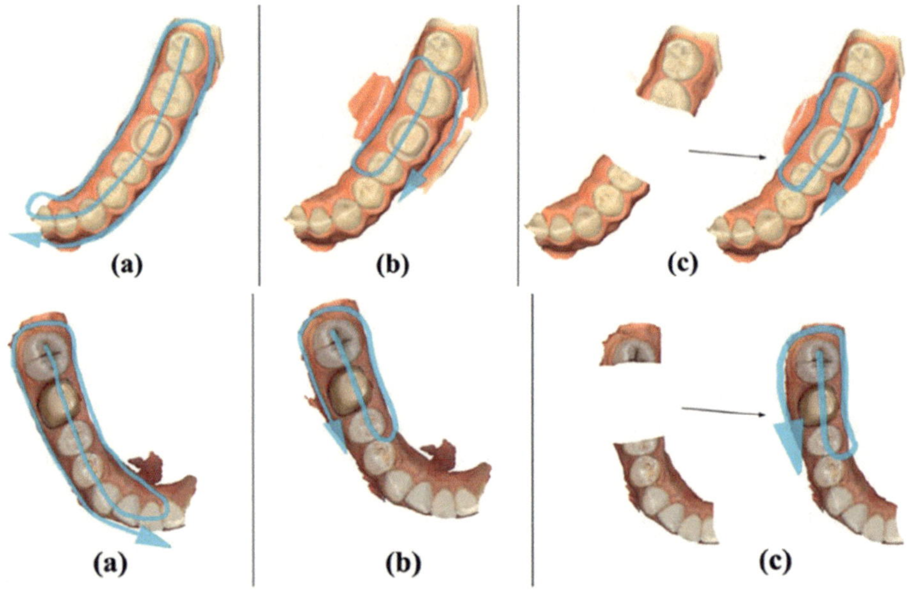

Figure 2.
Single uninterrupted scan (a), rescanning of the area of interest (b), and the deletion of the area of interest followed by a rescan (c).

but clinically insignificantly, the trueness outcomes were equivalent for both *in vivo* and *in vitro* scenarios [28].

3. Digital workflow for chairside smile design rehabilitation

After intraoral scanning, there are two options to send the: STL file *via* Internet to the dental laboratory, and then the dental technician will create the digital design, mill the restoration, or print it 3D, or the practician can make the design in office, with an adequate software and then finalize the restoration by milling or 3D printing.

There are several designs software designated for chairside restorations — CEREC (Dentsply Sirona), and Plan CAD Easy (Planmeca). The concept of same-day crown or same-day dentistry means that the dentist has the full control and responsibility from the case selection, to preparation, intraoral scanning, digital design, material selection, milling, and postprocessing of the restoration until the final cementation.

In order to make the final digital design, the dentist should make a careful examination and treatment planning for the future restoration. From veneers, inlays, onlays, crowns, and different minimally invasive restorations, such as tabletops, endo-crowns, and a multitude of single-unit restorations, can be designed with an *in office* software.

The following case reveals the importance of examination and planning when smile design rehabilitation is obtained with chairside CAD/CAM technology. A 42-year-old female patient presented for improving the appearance of her smile (**Figure 3**). When all the frontal teeth are involved, it is convenient to simulate the future smile design with the help of a digital smile design software (**Figure 4**). The color of the future restoration can be appreciated by combining traditional methods (tooth shade guide) and digital methods (spectrophotometers and software such as digital shade assistant (Ivoclar) **Figure 5**).

DOI: http://dx.doi.org/10.5772/intechopen.114090

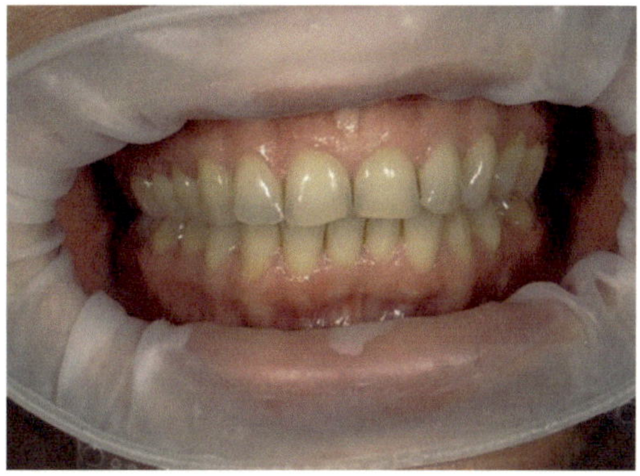

Figure 3.
Initial situation of the patient.

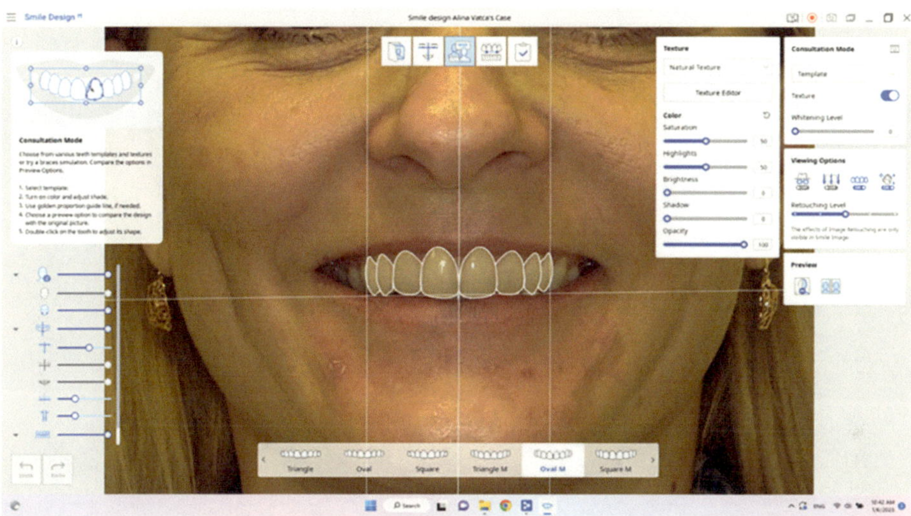

Figure 4.
Digital smile design (Medit).

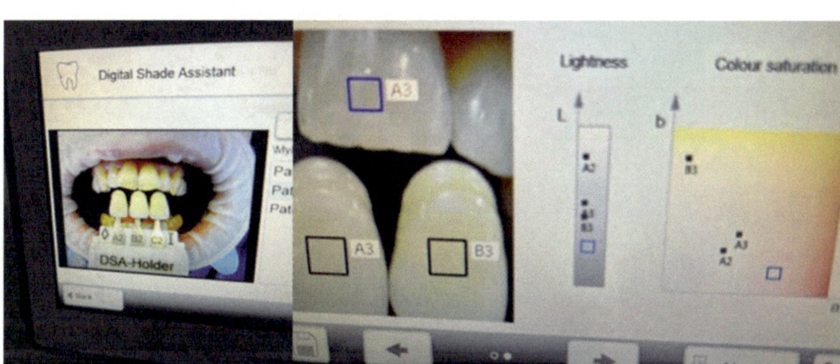

Figure 5.
Shade analysis with digital shade assistant (Programat CS6, Ivoclar).

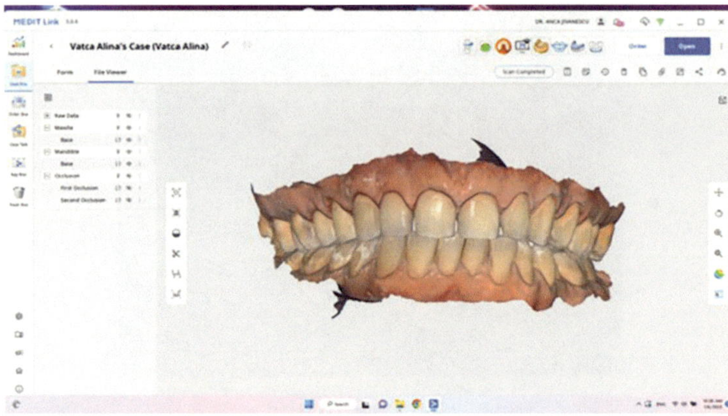

Figure 6.
Digital impression after teeth preparation.

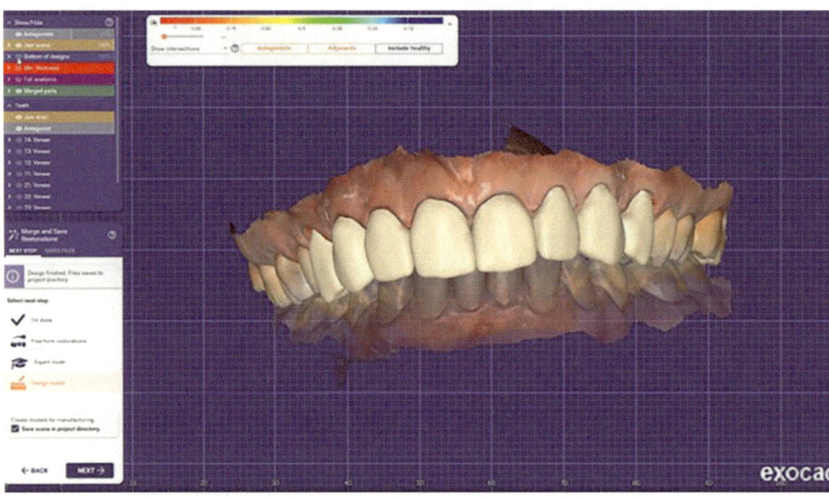

Figure 7.
Digital design for the eight veneers with EXOCAD software.

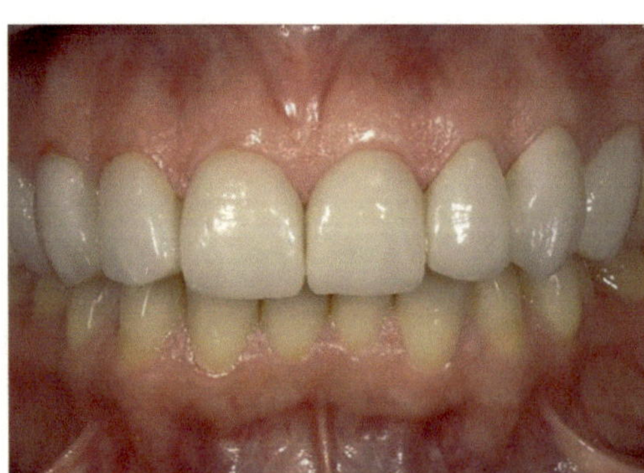

Figure 8.
Lithium disilicate (emax.CAD) veneers after cementation.

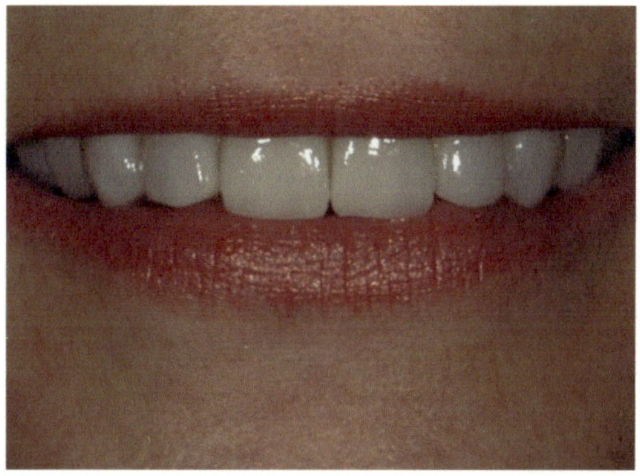

Figure 9.
The final smile of the patient.

After tooth preparation for eight veneers (from tooth 1.4. to 2.4.), an intraoral scanning was performed with Medit i700 (**Figure 6**). Then with a CAD software (exocad), the digital design for the eight veneers was performed (**Figure 7**), and send to the milling machine (Planmill 40, Planmeca). Eight veneers from lithium disilicate (emax. CAD) were milled and then bonded to the tooth structure with a precise adhesive protocol, using dual-cured resin cement (Variolink Esthetic, Ivoclar, Vivadent). (**Figure 8**). The final smile of the patient revealed the esthetic and functional improvement (**Figure 9**).

4. CAD/CAM equipment and materials used for prosthetic restorations

The first generation of CAD/CAM equipment was available on the market in the 1980s and could only be used to design and manufacture single ceramic restorations. Dental milling machines, usually integrated into bigger CAD/CAM systems are a real help for dental technicians or dentists design the restoration using CAD software, and CAM software creates the toolpaths that the milling machine needs to use for creating the restoration. Chairside milling machines are small devices intended for use in offices. Comparing these machines to their laboratory counterparts, they are frequently faster and smaller. Advancements in milling machine technology have led to a continuous improvement in the fit quality of digitally created dental restorations [29]. Chairside systems offer so many new options that they will inevitably become a standard feature of dental practices. Today's leading chairside systems employ a "full-digital workflow" to create a variety of prosthetic devices, including inlays/onlays, veneers, endo-crowns, bridges, crowns, and implant abutments, to mention only a few [4].

The clinicians can now choose from a variety of materials such as feldspathic, leucite ceramics, lithium disilicate glass-ceramics, resin, or hybrid materials. These materials can be classified using a variety of parameters such as resistance, composition, purpose, and manufacturing method [30]. These materials for chairside CAD/CAM systems are presented in blocks, which are delivered in a variety of color ranges and translucencies, exhibit qualities that are homogeneous, dense, and faultless, and provide highly esthetically pleasing restorations. However, surface characterization and color individualization can be completed before the firing for ceramic materials (**Figure 10**) [31, 32].

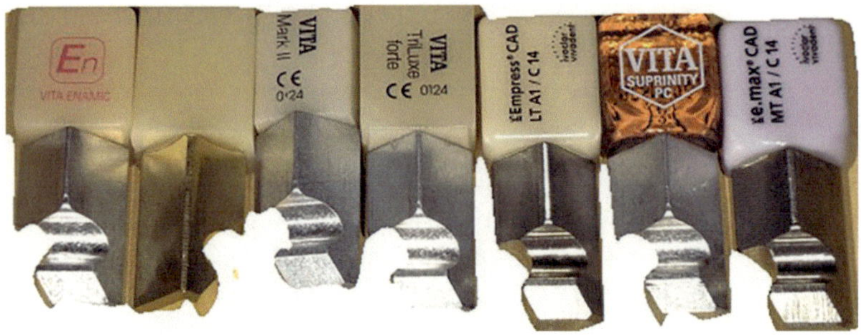

Figure 10.
Different ceramic and hybrid blocks for chairside milling machine (Planmill, Planmeca).

4.1 The classification of chairside CAD/CAM ceramic materials

From the perspective of composition and characteristics, CAD/CAM chairside ceramic materials can be categorized into four categories.

4.1.1 Feldspathic ceramics and leucite-reinforced ceramic blocks

The first generation of chairside CAD/CAM materials is represented by feldspathic ceramics (Vitablocs Mark II- Vita Zahnfabrik, CEREC Blocs - Dentsply Sirona,).

Prior to 1990, these materials were initially made available for commercial usage. They remained dominant in the market until the 2000s, and from a lifespan standpoint, they were also the most studied materials.

Feldspathic ceramics have a glassy phase predominance of between 55 and 70%, making them some of the most translucent and esthetically pleasing ceramic materials [33].

4.1.2 Lithium disilicates and zirconia-reinforced lithium silicates blocks

A significant advancement in the realm of fixed prostheses was the invention of glass ceramics with enhanced resistance qualities. In comparison to earlier glass ceramics, lithium disilicate (IPS e.max CAD Ivoclar Vivadent) was released in 2006 with a bending resistance exceeding 350 MPa.

Lithium disilicate is only provided in partially crystallized form (purple color) for the CAD/CAM method, where the block is made up of lithium metasilicate (Li_2SiO_3) and the remaining portion is made up of the crystallized nucleus of lithium disilicate ($Li_2Si_2O_5$), which provides a "soft" state (with a bending resistance of 140 MPa). This lessens the wear on the milling cutters and makes it easier to grind the block. The material needs to go through a two-stage fire cycle in a ceramic furnace for 10 minutes after milling to completely crystallize and change the metasilicate into lithium disilicate, which results in an increase in bending resistance over 440 MPa [34, 35].

Zirconia-reinforced lithium silicate (ZLS) is a newer generation of high-strength CAD/CAM ceramics that have been available since 2012. In ZLS, the glass matrix is reinforced with lithium silicate crystals that are 4–8 times smaller than those of lithium disilicate, and it is also given a 10% by weight tetragonal zirconia component to enhance its mechanical properties [36].

4.1.3 Zirconium oxide (zirconia)

Zirconium oxide or zirconia is a heterogeneous polycrystalline ceramic with exceptional mechanical characteristics (flexural strength 500–1200 MPa, elastic modulus 210 GPa); however, it is resistant to conventional acid etching techniques. It exhibits great biocompatibility both *in vivo* and *in vitro*, has lower plaque retention than titanium, and among the many integral ceramics, has the lowest rate of wear against the antagonist [37, 38].

The zirconia blocks for chairside CAD/CAM systems allow for simply soft machining processing of pre-sintered zirconia. Zirconia restorations are milled with a 25% oversize of the final volume, and the sinter process that follow will produce the perfect fit. This material can be used to make single crowns, implant abutments, and bridges with up to three parts by using chairside blocks [39, 40].

4.1.4 The hybrid ceramics or resin matrix ceramic materials

Hybrid ceramics are a brand-new class of CAD/CAM chairside materials that were created to combine the distinctive esthetic qualities of ceramic materials with the reduced fragility and greater fracture resistance of composite resins. A ceramic filler (up to 80% by weight) is coupled with a composite resin-like Bis-GMA, UDMA, UTMA, and Bis-EMA) in nanoceramic resin blocks made industrially by high-temperature and high-pressure processes. In the instance of polymer-infiltrated-ceramic network (PICN) blocks, composite resin (14% by bulk) has been industrially infused into the ceramic structure, which accounts for 86% of the block's bulk.

Hybrid ceramics have shown to be less difficult to mill and require no or fewer heat cycles. Additionally, they have good bending resistance and can still be employed at thinner thicknesses [41].

In the past 10 years, numerous novel components with greater mechanical characteristics have been created for CAD/CAM technology. The norms of dental care have greatly improved with the advent of new nanomaterials. Restorative dental science is thought to benefit greatly from nano-dentistry since it will enable tailored therapy [42, 43].

Dental composites' mechanical qualities have been enhanced using nanoparticles, which also strengthen bonds and reduce wear. Smaller particles can more effectively penetrate deeper lesions and lower the porosity of dental composite for increased toughness [44].

4.1.5 Acrylic resin

Polymethyl methacrylate (PMMA) based polymers are pre-polymerized without the addition of fillers and kept in storage until needed. Their cross-linked structure and chemical make-up determine their mechanical qualities primarily. The absence of voids and decreased shrinkage due to polymerization during mixing, packing, and setting have an important role in mechanical characteristics. A shortened chairside time can be used to create interim prostheses. Long-term temporary prosthesis could likewise be made using these PMMA CAD/CAM blocks.

4.2 The properties of chairside CAD/CAM materials

Clinical treatment results are directly correlated with the care taken to select the distinctive traits and features of the various types of CAD/CAM materials. Several variables, including material choice, restoration design, occlusion, and cementation, affect how well chairside restorations will succeed [45–47].

While the functional aspects of CAD/CAM materials have been extensively studied and implemented, there is an equally compelling need to focus on their esthetics. Esthetics play a pivotal role in several industries, including dentistry, where natural-looking restorations and prosthetics are in high demand [48–50].

4.2.1 Investigations on esthetic properties

The selection of a suitable material needs to match the natural tooth structure in terms of both mechanical properties and visual appearance, considering that oral restorations are exposed to various complex oral conditions during their lifetimes. Visual characteristics, such as color, texture, and translucency, are crucial for achieving a restoration that seamlessly blends with the surrounding natural teeth, providing a natural-looking smile.

One of the oral conditions that require special attention is the gastroesophageal reflux disease, which is characterized by regular regurgitations of gastric juice from the stomach into the oral cavity [51, 52]. A significant need for intraoral use and a deciding factor when selecting the kind of restoration is dental materials' resistance to chemical deterioration. Acid concentration, immersion time, and temperature, all these parameters affect the *in vitro* simulation of acid on the surface of dental ceramics [51]. Several studies performed in Department of Prosthodontics; Faculty of Dentistry Timisoara (TADERP Research Center) involved the consequences of oral conditions with this pathology on the properties of these new materials.

A significant need for intraoral use and a deciding factor when selecting the kind of restoration is dental materials' resistance to chemical deterioration. Acid concentration, immersion time, and temperature, all these parameters affect the *in vitro* simulation of acid on the surface of dental ceramics [52–55]. It can be inferred from other study publications in the literature that there is not a lot of agreement on how to simulate stomach acid and how long it takes to replicate it in an *in vivo* model. The usage of 4% acetic acid and an exposure length of 16 hours at 8°C is equivalent to 2 years of clinical exposure, according to ISO standard 6872, which deals with the solubility test for dental materials [48].

Several studies performed in Department of Prosthodontics; Faculty of Dentistry Timisoara (TADERP Research Center) involved the consequences of oral conditions with this pathology on the properties of these new materials. In one study, it was shown that for all tested monolithic materials, scanning electron microscopy revealed noticeable alterations to the material's topography after simulated gastric acid exposure for feldspathic ceramic, nanoceramic resin, hybrid ceramic, and leucite-reinforced glass ceramic. Triluxe Forte (VITA Zahnfabrik- Bad Säckingen, Germany), Cerasmart (GC Europe), Enamic (VITA Zahnfabrik- Bad Säckingen, Germany), and Empress CAD (Ivoclar, Schaan, Liechtenstein) were the tested materials. Using scanning electron microscopy, their microhardness, surface roughness, translucency, and surface morphology were examined both before and after exposure to simulated stomach acid liquid. The results of this investigation revealed that Triluxe Forte was the CAD-CAM monolithic restorative material that underwent the most significant modifications following exposure to a gastric acid simulation. The Cerasmart monolithic restorative material, however, was found to be least impacted following a simulation of exposure to gastric acid [56].

Another *in vitro* investigation into the color stability of chairside CAD/CAM ceramic blocks made of leucitic, feldspathic, and disilicate following exposure to common liquids was performed. According to the study's findings, all materials showed color changes after being submerged in red wine that was just barely above the thresholds for perceptibility and acceptability. The feldspathic CAD/CAM ceramic blocks showed the most notable color changes after being submerged in coffee. Within the bounds of this study's limitations, it may be inferred that typical beverages may have an impact on the CAD/CAM ceramic blocks' color stability, which may jeopardize the esthetics of the restorations [57].

4.2.2 Investigations on mechanical properties

The mechanical characteristics of CAD/CAM materials require a special consideration. For researchers and physicians understanding a restorative material's mechanical characteristics is crucial because significant fracturing of these materials has been identified as the primary reason of failure. One *in vitro* study evaluated the fracture resistance and surface of full contour Vita Enamic CAD/CAM crowns with different thicknesses [58]. According to the study's findings, crowns with a 1.5 mm thickness had a larger compression load than crowns with a 0.5 or 1.0 mm thickness. The fracture loads in the groups with occlusal thicknesses of 0.5 and 1.0 mm did not differ significantly.

In contrast to stiffer materials such as high translucency zirconia and zirconia-reinforced glass ceramic, PINC distributes more stress to the abutment [59, 60]. A thicker restorative material will increase the restoration's fracture resistance, according to some researchers who observed that prolonged tooth preparation will damage the remaining tooth structure and cause permanent failure [61–64]. The findings of this study show that, regardless of the thickness of the crown, restored teeth using PICN CAD/CAM crowns can attain compression load values between 700 and 2500 N. Even in bruxism patients who are developing masticatory forces of 780 to 1120 N during mastication, these values are higher than the human masticatory forces (600–800 N). The conclusion was that the force generated by the physiologic masticatory process was less than the load placed on polymer-infiltrated ceramic network restorations. For posterior region restorations, CAD/CAM hybrid ceramic materials can offer enough fracture strength and load capacity.

The ideal dental restoration should present perfect marginal adaptation, biocompatibility with oral environment, esthetics, and long-term mechanical strength. Another study regarding the compressive strength evaluation of different CAD/CAM materials takes into consideration the oral conditions previously mentioned as crucial when choosing the appropriate material for a long-term rehabilitation case. Thin occlusal veneers processed from various CAD/CAM blocks can be an ideal alternative to restore tooth wear because of the development of new adhesive materials and procedures [63]. The current study's goal was to evaluate the compressive strength of thin occlusal veneers manufactured of three distinct CAD/CAM supplies (Cerasmart, Straumann Nice, and Tetric CAD) before and after they were immersed in acidic artificial saliva. The results of the current study demonstrated that all three CAD/CAM restorative material types—nanoceramic, glass ceramic, and resin composite—are appropriate alternatives for patients who have tooth wear even when they have a 0.5 mm thin thickness and follow the proper cementation technique. When compared to occlusal veneers that were immersed in artificial saliva that was acidic and/or subjected to temperature cycling, the studied 0.5 mm thick occlusal veneers manufactured from CAD/CAM restorative materials showed higher compressive loads. Even the specimens that had been subjected to artificial saliva that was acidic had values that were higher than both normal and parafunctional bite forces. The composition of a restorative material generally determines its mechanical strength, although endogenous and/or exogenous variables (such as acidic foods or beverages, stomach acid, water sorption, cariogenic biofilm, or salivary enzymes) may also have an impact through material deterioration [64–66]. Due to the low pH level, endogenous acids deteriorate both dental structure and restoration [67]. The most recent composites and ceramic hybrid materials allow milling surfaces to be created even at a thin thickness, preserving the residual tooth structure. Comparable to reinforced ceramics, occlusal veneers (tabletops) made of composite resin blocks have superior fatigue resistance [68].

The findings of various investigations on the partial coverage of ceramic restorations are inconclusive. Even though most manufacturers advise posterior ceramic restorations to have a minimum thickness of 1.5 mm, several research studies have examined ceramic restorations with a thickness of 1.0 mm or even less that have excellent long-term clinical results [68–74].

The micro-shear bond strength of glass-ceramic materials, such as lithium disilicate ceramic, leucite-reinforced ceramic, and a hybrid ceramic, was examined in a different study [75]. The vitreous component, a crucial element in adhesive cementation, is a characteristic of both ceramic materials and hybrid ceramics. Adhesive cementation needs both chemical and micromechanical retention [76–78]. Resin cement have a better strength than self-adhesive cement, and they are typically dual-cured to ensure appropriate polymerization [79, 80]. Ceramic restorations and dentine need to have their surfaces pre-treated before cementation to obtain optimal adhesion and chemical and micromechanical retention [81–83]. When HF acid gets applied to a ceramic surface, the silica matrix reacts, causing the surface layer of the glassy matrix including silica, silicates, and leucite crystals to dissolve and be removed. According to the composition of the ceramics and the distribution of their crystalline and vitreous phases, each ceramic material exhibits a unique, original etching design. With an increased geometrical pattern in the ceramic structure, HF acid increases the bond strength between the restoration and adhesive, as well as the wettability and surface energy of the substrate. It also leaves behind a surface that is ready for the luting material to penetrate and diffuse into [84–86]. The results of our study demonstrated that a longer HF acid etching time caused more ceramic to dissolve, which produced a stronger link to resin cement. Still, there was not much of variation between the 30 and 60 s values, thus it was decided that for lithium disilicate, it was best to use either a higher acid concentration with the manufacturer-recommended period or a longer time [75].

4.2.3 Research on the biocompatibility of CAD/CAM materials

Biocompatibility is an important aspect of ceramic materials. According to literature, ceramic materials have greater biocompatibility and cell response compared to polymers in terms of their biocompatibility. In the past 10 years, numerous enhanced materials with superior mechanical properties have been created for CAD/CAM technology [45, 86–93].

A recent study was focused on the biocompatibility and sustainability of human fibroblasts and keratinocyte cells on ceramic and composite CAD/CAM materials [81]. For this purpose, three ceramic and composite CAD/CAM materials (Cerasmart

(CS)—nanoceramic resin; Straumann Nice (SN)—glass ceramic; and Tetric CAD (TC)—composite resin) from various manufacturers were subjected to testing.

There are not many studies that have been documented in the scientific literature about the biocompatibility of these kinds of CAD/CAM restorative materials. For instance, a recent study provided information on the biocompatibility and sustainability of three types of ceramics: Vita Enamic (EN), Cerasmart (CS), and Brilliant Crios (BC). Transmission electron microscopy (TEM) measurements of surface roughness, biofilm formation, cytotoxicity, genotoxicity, and cellular alterations led the scientists to the conclusion that there was no appreciable variation in surface roughness between the examined CAD/CAM blocks. Furthermore, there is no link between surface roughness and the development of biofilms. When cytotoxicity was considered, BC displayed the highest values, followed by CS and EN. As a result, EN was determined to be the evaluated materials' most biocompatible substance [94]. A unique lithium silicate glass ceramic was created and developed by Daguano and colleagues, who also tested its biocompatibility *in vitro*. In contrast to other glass ceramics that already exist in the same family, the new lithia-silica glass ceramic is bioactive. This is the most significant discovery. It encouraged the formation of a bone-like matrix in MG-63 cells, which may be crucial for bone regeneration in and dental applications. Additionally, it promoted cell adhesion and growth [95]. As pointed in the preciouses' studies, long-term oral exposure to the tooth-restoration hybrid necessitates consideration of the impact of intrinsic and extrinsic substances on these surfaces. Because acid from the stomach commonly refluxes into the or mouth cavity, patients with gastroesophageal reflux are the most vulnerable in this circumstance [51].

Considering the aforementioned information, the objective of our study was to examine the early response and biocompatibility of three dental materials when they encountered human keratinocyte and gingival fibroblast cells. To determine whether acidic artificial saliva could affect the biocompatibility of restorative materials when in contact with living organisms, it was intended to look at how the three different CAD/CAM restorative materials would differ in composition and structure in an acidic environment. Regarding biological activity, it was discovered how cytotoxic two different types of typical human cell lines—fibroblasts (BJ) and keratinocytes (HaCaT)—to three restorative materials—Cerasmart—CS, Straumann Nice—SN, and Tetric CAD—TC—were [93]. The results indicated that the examined samples can be classified as slightly cytotoxic and noncytotoxic in terms of the proliferation of human keratinocytes, except for SN_B, which recorded a reduced mitochondrial activity (about 50%). In terms of NO production, keratinocytes produced somewhat more NO than fibroblasts, while fibroblasts produced NO at a decreased rate that was cut to half. Determining cell oxidative stress on the nitric route is, therefore, not possible with the examined materials. When the fibroblast cells were set up on each compact dental material (CS, SN, and TC), they became attached and spread out, preferring the TC material. Yet when the fibroblast cells were exposed to the acidic environment of each material and tested, they ought to suffer the most [96].

5. Conclusion

- Chairside CAD/CAM restorative materials have many advantages such as their ease of preparation, polishing, reparability, and future studies, examining the substances released from CAD/CAM restorative materials and their effects will be significant.

- Even if there are many advantages of using the digital approach, there are certain factors that can influence the accuracy of a digital impression. The ambient light, the fluid isolation, scanning pattern and distance, or the rescanning of the same surface, all these variables can lead to a less accurate digital impression.
- Regarding the ambient light, there is no consensus regarding the ideal lighting conditions since different studies presented different results, but it is safe to assume that high illumination sources may oversaturate the scanned areas leading to artifacts in the digital model.
- Rescanning of an area is to be avoided. However, there are mixed reports regarding its influence in the accuracy of a scan.
- Furthermore, no single study has produced conclusive results about the best scanning pattern, and the majority of research indicates that the scanning technique has a major impact on scanning accuracy, even though other studies indicate that, with the scanners available today, the scanning pattern has no effect on the quality of the digital impression.
- The accuracy of a digital impression can be affected by the distance between the tip of the IOS and the recorded surface; maintaining approximately 5–10 mm can generate accurate digital models.
- The materials used in the digital workflow also play a key role in the success of the prosthetic treatments.
- Knowing the mechanical strength and esthetical properties of each class is essential for predictable treatments.
- While feldspathic ceramics are used mainly in the anterior arch due to their inferior strength and high esthetics, lithium disilicate and zirconia are well suited to withstand the occlusal loads of the posterior area.
- Hybrid ceramics are also an option presenting good flexural resistance and allow for more conservative treatments.

Author details

Anca Jivanescu, Ille Codruta* and Raul Rotar
Faculty of Dentistry, Department of Prosthodontics, Victor Babes University of Medicine and Pharmacy, Timisoara, Romania

*Address all correspondence to: ille.codruta@umft.ro

References

[1] Mangano F, Shibli JA, Fortin T. Digital dentistry. New Materials and Techniques. 2016;**2016**:5261247. DOI: 10.1155/2016/5261247

[2] Murdoch-Kinch CA, McLean ME. Minimally invasive dentistry. The Journal of the American Dental Association. 2003;**134**(1):87-95, ISSN 00028177. DOI: 10.14219/jada.archive.2003.0021. Available from: https://www.sciencedirect.com/science/article/pii/S0002817714619577

[3] Davidowitz G, Kotick PG. The use of CAD/CAM in dentistry. Dental Clinics of North America. 2011;**55**(3):559-570, ix

[4] Mörmann WHBM. State of the art of CAD-CAM restorations: 20 years of CEREC. In: Quintessence Books. 1st ed. Berlin: Quintessence Publishing Co Ltd; 2006. pp. 1-8

[5] Ueda Y, Yamaguchi T. History of and current situation regarding dental CAD/CAM systems and future perspectives. Journal of Dental Sciences. 2017;**38**:104-110

[6] Rekow ED. Digital dentistry: The new state of the art—is it disruptive or destructive? Dental Materials. 2020;**36**:9-24

[7] Tabesh M, Nejatidanesh F, Savabi G, Davoudi A, Savabi O, Mirmohammadi H. Marginal adaptation of zirconia complete coverage fixed dental restorations made from digital scans or conventional impressions: A systematic review and meta-analysis. The Journal of Prosthetic Dentistry. 2021;**125**:603-610

[8] Diker B, Tak Ö. Accuracy of six intraoral scanners for scanning complete-arch and 4-unit fixed partial dentures: An *in vitro* study. The Journal of Prosthetic Dentistry. 2021;**128**(2):187-194

[9] Abduo J, Elseyoufi M. Accuracy of intraoral scanners: A systematic review of influencing factors. The European Journal of Prosthodontics and Restorative Dentistry. 2018;**26**(3):101-121

[10] Arakida T, Kanazawa M, Iwaki M, Suzuki T, Minakuchi S. Evaluating the influence of ambient light on scanning trueness, precision, and time of intra oral scanner. Journal of Prosthodontic Research. 2018;**62**(3):324-329

[11] Gerbino S, Del Giudice DM, Staiano G, Lanzotti A, Martorelli M. On the influence of scanning factors on the laser scanner-based 3D inspection process. International Journal of Advanced Manufacturing Technology. 2016;**84**:1787-1799

[12] Jivanescu A, Faur AB, Rotar RN. Can dental office lighting intensity conditions influence the accuracy of intraoral scanning? Scanning. 2021;**27**(2021):9980590. DOI: 10.1155/2021/9980590

[13] Holroyd M, Lawrence J. An analysis of using high-frequency sinusoidal illumination to measure the 3D shape of translucent objects. In: Proceedings of the IEEE Computer Society Conference on Computer Vision and Pattern Recognition. 2011. pp. 2985-2991. DOI: 10.1109/CVPR.2011.5995536

[14] Li H, Lyu P, Wang Y, Sun Y. Influence of object translucency on the scanning accuracy of a powder-free intraoral scanner: A laboratory study. The Journal of Prosthetic Dentistry. 2017;**117**(1):93-101

[15] Kurz M, Attin T, Mehl A. Influence of material surface on the scanning error of a powder-free 3D measuring system. Clinical Oral Investigations. 2015;**19**(8):2035-2043

[16] Medina-Sotomayor P, Pascual MA, Camps AI. Accuracy of four digital scanners according to scanning strategy in complete-arch impressions. PLoS ONE. 2018;**13**(9):e0202916. DOI: 10.1371/journal.pone.0202916

[17] Renne W, Ludlow M, Fryml J, Schurch Z, Mennito A, Kessler R, et al. Evaluation of the accuracy of 7 digital scanners: An *in vitro* analysis based on 3-dimensional comparisons. The Journal of Prosthetic Dentistry [Internet]. 2017;**118**(1):36-42. DOI: 10.1016/j.prosdent.2016.09.024

[18] Oh KC, Park J, Moon HS. Effects of scanning strategy and scanner type on the accuracy of intraoral scans: A new approach for assessing the accuracy of scanned data. Journal of Prosthodontics. 2020;**29**(6):518-523

[19] Motel C, Kirchner E, Adler W, Wichmann M, Matta RE. Impact of different scan bodies and scan strategies on the accuracy of digital implant impressions assessed with an intraoral scanner: An *in vitro* study. Journal of Prosthodontics. 2020;**29**(4):309-314

[20] Rotar RN, Faur AB, Pop D, Jivanescu A. Scanning distance influence on the intraoral scanning accuracy-an *in vitro* study. Materials (Basel). 2022;**15**(9):3061. DOI: 10.3390/ma15093061

[21] Güth JF, Wallbach J, Stimmelmayr M, Gernet W, Beuer F, Edelhoff D. Computer-aided evaluation of preparations for CAD/CAM-fabricated all-ceramic crowns. Clinical Oral Investigations. 2013;**17**(5):1389-1395

[22] Carbajal Mejía JB, Wakabayashi K, Nakamura T, Yatani H. Influence of abutment tooth geometry on the accuracy of conventional and digital methods of obtaining dental impressions. The Journal of Prosthetic Dentistry [Internet]. 2017;**118**(3):392-399. Available from: http://www.sciencedirect.com/science/article/pii/S002239131630600X

[23] Beuer F, Aggstaller H, Richter J, Edelhoff D, Gernet W. Influence of preparation angle on marginal and internal fit of CAD/CAM-fabricated zirconia crown copings. Quintessence International (Berl). 2009;**40**(3):243-250

[24] Song J, Kim M. Accuracy on scanned images of full arch models with orthodontic brackets by various intraoral scanners in the presence of artificial saliva. BioMed Research International. 2020;**2020**:2920804

[25] Schubert O, Erdelt KJ, Tittenhofer R, Hajtó J, Bergmann A, Güth JF. Influence of intraoral scanning on the quality of preparations for all-ceramic single crowns. Clinical Oral Investigations. 2020;**24**(12):4511-4518

[26] Gómez-Polo M, Piedra-Cascón W, Methani MM, Quesada-Olmo N, Farjas-Abadia M, Revilla-León M. Influence of rescanning mesh holes and stitching procedures on the complete-arch scanning accuracy of an intraoral scanner: An *in vitro* study. Journal of Dentistry. 2021;**110**:103690

[27] Ali IE, Hattori M, Sumita YI, Wakabayashi N. Effect of cut-out rescan procedures on the accuracy of an intraoral scanner used for digitizing an ear model: An *in vitro* study. Journal of Prosthodontics. 2022;**32**(6):527-533

[28] Faur AB, Rotar RN, Adam D, Jivănescu A. Rescanning of digital

impressions' mesh holes: *In vivo* and *in vitro* accuracy evaluation of three different scanning protocols. Applied Sciences. 2023;**13**:2867. DOI: 10.3390/app13052867

[29] Makhija SK, Lawson NC, Gilbert GH, Litaker MS, McClelland JA, Louis DR, et al. Dentist material selection for single-unit crowns: Findings from the National Dental Practice-based research network. Journal of Dentistry. 2016;**55**:40-47, ISSN 0300-5712,. DOI: 10.1016/j.jdent.2016.09.010

[30] Van Noort R. The future of dental devices is digital. Dental Materials. 2012;**28**(1):3-12

[31] Fasbinder DJ. Materials for chairside CAD/CAM restorations. The Compendium of Continuing Education in Dentistry. 2010;**31**:702-704, 706, 708

[32] Vichi A, Carrabba M, Paravina R, Ferrari M. Translucency of ceramic materials for CEREC CAD/CAM system. Journal of Esthetic and Restorative Dentistry. 2014;**26**:224-231

[33] Tysowsky GW. The science behind lithium disilicate: A metal-free alternative. Dentistry Today. 2009;**28**:112-113

[34] Lien W, Roberts HW, Platt JA, Vandewalle KS, Hill TJ, Chu TM. Microstructural evolution and physical behaviour of a lithium disilicate glass-ceramic. Dental Materials. 2015;**31**:928-940

[35] Gehrt M, Wolfart S, Rafai N, Reich S, Edelhoff D. Clinical results of lithium disilicated crown after up to 9 years of service. Clinical Oral Investigations. 2013;**17**:275-284

[36] Manjot A. Recent advances in composite CAD/CAM blocks. The International Journal of Esthetic Dentistry. 2016;**11**:275-280

[37] Muhammad S, Zafar A, Alnazzawi A, Alrahabi M, Fareed AM, Najeeb S, et al. Nanotechnology and Nanomaterials in Dentistry, Advanced Dental Biomaterials. Sawston, United Kingdom: Woodhead Publishing; 2019. pp. 477-505. ISBN 9780081024768. DOI: 10.1016/B978-0-08-102476-8.00018-9

[38] Subramani K, Ahmed W, Hartsfield JK. Nanobiomaterials in Clinical Dentistry. Norwich: William Andrew; 2012

[39] Mok ZH, Proctor G, Thanou M. Emerging nanomaterials for dental treatments. Emerging Topics in Life Sciences. 2020;**4**(6):613-625. DOI: 10.1042/ETLS20200195

[40] Zarone F, Russo S, Sorrentino R. From porcelain-fused to metal to zirconia: Clinical and experimental considerations. Dental Materials. 2011;**87**:83-96

[41] Denry I, Kelly JR. State of the art of zirconia for dental applications. Dental Materials. 2008;**24**:299-307

[42] Nakashima J, Taira Y, Sawase T. In vitro wear of four ceramic materials and human enamel on enamel antagonist. European Journal of Oral Sciences. 2016;**124**:295-300

[43] Jivanescu A. Protetica dentara in era digitala. Timisoara: Editura Eurobit; 2019

[44] Marchesi G, Camurri Piloni A, Nicolin V, Turco G, Di Lenarda R. Chairside CAD/CAM materials: Current trends of clinical uses. Biology. 2021;**10**:1170. DOI: 10.3390/biology10111170

[45] Curtis AR, Shortall AC, Marquis PM, Palin WM. Water uptake and strength

characteristics of a nanofilled resin-basedcomposite. Journal of Dentistry. 2008;**36**:186-193

[46] Kim YS, Kwon HK, Kim BI. Effect of nano-carbonate apatite to prevent restain after dental bleaching *in vitro*. Journal of Dentistry. 2011;**39**:636-642

[47] Chen C, Trindade FZ, de Jager N, Kleverlaan CJ, Feilzer AJ. The fracture resistance of a CAD/CAM resin Nano ceramic (RNC) and a CAD ceramic at different thicknesses. Dental Materials. 2014;**30**:954-962

[48] Alves PB, Brandt WC, Neves AC, Gonçalves Cunha L. Silva-Concilio, mechanical properties of direct and indirect composites after storage for 24 h and 10 months. European Journal of Dentistry. 2013;7:117-122

[49] Belli R, Geinzer E, Muschweck A, Petschelt A, Lohbauer U. Mechanical fatigue degradation of ceramics versus resin composites for dental restorations. Dental Materials. 2014;**30**:424-432

[50] Aldamaty MF, Haggag KM, Othman HI. Effect of simulated gastric acid on surface roughness of different monolithic ceramics. Al-Azhar Journal of Dental Science. 2020;**23**:327-334

[51] El-Serag HB, Sweet S, Winchester CC, Dent J. Update on the epidemiology of gastro-oesophageal reflux disease: A systematic review. Gut. 2014;**63**:871-880

[52] Sulaiman TA, Abdulmajeed AA, Shahramian K, Hupa L, Donovan TE, Vallittu P, et al. Impact of gastric acidic challenge on surface topography and optical properties of monolithic zirconia. Dental Materials. 2015;**31**:1445-1452

[53] Cruz MEM, Simoes R, Martins SB, Trinidade FZ, Dovigo LN, Fonseca RG. Influence of simulated gastric juice on surface characteristics of CAD-CAM monolithic materials. The Journal of Prosthetic Dentistry. 2020;**123**:483-490

[54] Pîrvulescu IL, Pop D, Moacă E-A, Mihali C-V, Ille C, Jivănescu A. Effects of simulated gastric acid exposure on surface topography, mechanical and optical features of commercial CAD/CAM ceramic blocks. Applied Sciences. 2021;**11**:8703. DOI: 10.3390/app11188703

[55] Pîrvulescu I, Ille C, Rotar R, Goguță L, Cîrligeriu L, Jivănescu A. Color changes of different CAD/CAM blocks after immersion in usual beverages. RJOR. January-March 2021;**13**(1)

[56] Avram L, Goguta L, Galatanu S-V, Opris C, Ille C, Jivanescu A. Material thickness influence on fracture load of polymer infiltrated ceramic network CAD/CAM restorations. Materiale Plastice. 2021;**119**:104485, Available from: https://revmaterialeplastice.ro . DOI: 10.37358/mat.plast.1964

[57] de Oliveira Dal Piva AM, Tribst JPM, Jalkh EBB, Anami LC, Bonfante EA, Bottino MA. Minimal tooth preparation for posterior monolithic ceramic crowns: Effect on the mechanical behavior, reliability and translucency. Dental Materials. 2021;**37**(3):e140-e150. DOI: 10.1016/j.dental.2020.11.001

[58] Arm S, Al-Ani M, Alrawi t. AL-Edressi G. An *in-vitro* comparison of fracture resistance of three CAD/CAM ceramic materials for fabricating veneer. The Saudi Dental Journal. 2020;**33**(7):745-752. DOI: 10.1016/j.sdentj.2020.03.013

[59] Luekiatpaisarn J, Leevailoj C. Fracture resistance of occlusal ceramic and composite molar onlay comparing to lithium disilicate molar crown. The Journal of the Dental Association

of Thailand. 2019;**69**(1):92-100. DOI: 10.14456/jdat.2019.11

[60] Xu Z, Yu P, Arola DD, Min J, Gao S. A comparative study on the wear behavior of a polymer infiltrated ceramic network (PICN) material and tooth enamel. Dental Materials. 2017;**33**(12):1351-1361. DOI: 10.1016/j.dental.2017.08.190

[61] Jun SK, Kim DA, Goo HJ, Lee HH. Investigation of the correlation between the different mechanical properties of resin composites. Dental Materials Journal. 2013;**32**:48-57

[62] Seow WK, Thong KM. Erosive effects of common beverages on extracted premolar teeth. Australian Dental Journal. 2005;**50**:173-178

[63] Wongkhantee S, Patanapiradej V, Maneenut C, Tantbirojn D. Effect of acidic food and drinks on surface hardness of enamel, dentine, and tooth-colored filling materials. Journal of Dentistry. 2006;**34**:214-220

[64] Larsen IB, Munksgaard EC. Effect of human saliva on surface degradation of composite resins. Scandinavian Journal of Dental Research. 1991;**99**:254-261

[65] Turssi CP, Hara AT, de Magalhaes CS, Campos Serra M, Rodrigues AL Jr. Influence of storage regime prior to abrasion on surface topography of restorative materials. Journal of Biomedical Materials Research. Part B, Applied Biomaterials. 2003;**65**:227-232

[66] Johnson AC, Versluis A, Tantbirojn D, Ahuja S. Fracture strength of CAD/CAM composite and composite-ceramic occlusal veneers. Journal of Prosthodontic Research. 2014;**58**(2):107-114

[67] Guess PC, Schultheis S, Wolkewitz M, Zhang Y, Strub JR. Influence of preparation design and ceramic thicknesses on fracture resistance and failure modes of premolar partial coverage restorations. The Journal of Prosthetic Dentistry. 2013;**110**(4):264-273

[68] Sasse M, Krummel A, Klosa K, Kern M. Influence of restoration thickness and dental bonding surface on the fracture resistance of full-coverage occlusal veneers made from lithium disilicate ceramic. Dental Materials. 2015;**31**(8):907-915

[69] Albelasy E, Hamama HH, Tsoi JKH, Mahmoud SH. Influence of material type, thickness and storage on fracture resistance of CAD/CAM occlusal veneers. Journal of the Mechanical Behavior of Biomedical Materials. 2021;**119**:104485-104494

[70] Andrade JP, Stona D, Bittencourt HR, Borges GA, Burnett LHJ, Spohr AM. Effect of different computer-aided design/computer aided manufacturing (CAD/CAM) materials and thicknesses on the fracture resistance of occlusal veneers. Operative Dentistry. 2018;**43**(5):539-548

[71] Singhatanadgit W, Junkaew P, Singhatanadgid P. Effect of bidirectional loading on contact and force characteristics under a newly developed masticatory simulator with a dual-direction loading system. Dental Materials Journal. 2016;**35**(6):952-961

[72] Ille C, Moacă EA, Pop D, Goguță L, Opriș C, Pîrvulescu IL, et al. Compressive strength evaluation of thin occlusal veneers from different CAD/CAM materials, before and after acidic saliva exposure. Odontology. 2022;**111**(2):360-374. DOI: 10.1007/s10266-022-00741-5

[73] Avram LT, Galațanu S-V, Opriș C, Pop C, Jivănescu A. Effect of different etching times with hydrofluoric acid on

the bond strength of CAD/CAM ceramic material. Materials. 2022;**15**:7071. DOI: 10.3390/ma15207071

[74] Bebsh M, Haimeur A, França R. The effect of different surface treatments on the micromorphology and the roughness of four dental CAD/CAM lithium silicate-based glass-ceramics. Ceramics. 2021;**4**:467-475

[75] Nogueira IDO, de Oliveira PFG, Magno MB, Ferreira DMTP, Maia LC, Rabello T. Does the application of an adhesive layer improve the bond strength of etched and silanized glass-ceramics to resin-based materials? A systematic review and meta-analysis. The Journal of Prosthetic Dentistry. 2021;**125**(1):56-64

[76] Fernandes VVB Jr, Oliani MG, Nogueira L Jr, Silva JMF, Araújo RM. Analysis and comparison of different bond strength tests. JSM Dentistry. 2016;**4**:1076

[77] Aldhafyan M, Silikas N, Watts DC. Influence of curing modes on thermal stability, hardness development and network integrity of dual-cure resin cements. Dental Materials. 2021;**37**:1854-1864

[78] Rani S, Kansal R, Kumar M, Kumar S, Issar G. Comparative evaluation of shear bond strength of newer resin cement (RelyX ultimate and RelyX U200) to lithium disilicate and zirconia ceramics as influenced by thermocycling. Contemporary Clinical Dentistry. 2018;**9**:601-606

[79] Ustun S, Ayaz EA. Effect of different cement systems and aging on the bond strength of chairside CAD-CAM ceramics. The Journal of Prosthetic Dentistry. 2021;**125**:334-339

[80] Lanza MDS, Vasconcellos WA, De Miranda GLP, Peixoto RTRDC, Lanza LD. Different bonding agents effect on adhesive bond strength: Lithium disilicate glass ceramic. Revista de Odontologia da UNESP. 2020;**49**:e20200020

[81] Wong ACH, Tian T, Tsoi JKH, Burrow MF, Matinlinna JP. Aspects of adhesion tests on resin–glass ceramic bonding. Dental Materials. 2017;**33**:1045-1055

[82] Yanakiev S, Yordanov B, Marinova-Takorova M, Filaretova Y. Hydrofluoric acid etching patterns and surface morphology of three silica-based ceramic materials. Journal of IMAB – Annual Proceeding (Scientific Papers). 2022;**28**:4325-4329

[83] Günal-Abduljalil B, Önöral Ö, Ongun S. Micro-shear bond strengths of resin-matrix ceramics subjected to different surface conditioning strategies with or without coupling agent application. Journal of Advanced Prosthodontics. 2021;**13**:180-190

[84] Puppin-Rontani J, Sundfeld D, Costa A, Correr A, Borges G, Sinhoreti M, et al. Effect of hydrofluoric acid concentration and etching time on bond strength to lithium disilicate glass ceramic. Operative Dentistry. 2017;**42**:606-615

[85] Schmalz G, Galler KM. Biocompatibility of biomaterials—Lessons learned and considerations for the design of novel materials. Dental Materials. 2017;**33**:382-393

[86] Rizo-Gorrita M, Herráez-Galindo C, Torres-Lagares D, Serrera-Figallo M-Á, Gutiérre-Pérez J-L. Biocompatibility of polymer and ceramic CAD/CAM materials with human gingival fibroblasts (HGFs). Polymers. 2019;**11**:1446

[87] Sonmez N, Gultekin P, Turp V, Akgungor G, Sen D, Mijiritsky E. Evaluation of five CAD/CAM materials by microstructural characterization and mechanical tests: A comparative *in vitro* study. BMC Oral Health. 2018;**18**:5

[88] Blackburn C, Rask H, Awada A. Mechanical properties of resin-ceramic CAD-CAM materials after accelerated aging. The Journal of Prosthetic Dentistry. 2018;**119**:954-958

[89] Giordano R. Materials for chairside CAD/CAM-produced restorations. Journal of the American Dental Association (1939). 2006;**137**(Suppl. 1):14S-21S

[90] D'Arcangelo C, Vanini L, Rondoni GD, De Angelis F. Wear properties of dental ceramics and porcelains compared with human enamel. The Journal of Prosthetic Dentistry. 2016;**115**:350-355

[91] Ankyu S, Nakamura K, Harada A, Hong G, Kanno T, Niwano Y, et al. Fatigue analysis of computer-aided design/computer-aided manufacturing resin-based composite vs. lithium disilicate glass-ceramic. European Journal of Oral Sciences. 2016;**124**:387-395

[92] Grzebieluch W, Mikulewicz M, Kaczmarek U. Resin composite materials for chairside CAD/CAM restorations: A comparison of selected mechanical properties. Journal of Healthcare Engineering. 2021;**2021**:8828954

[93] Holban A-M, Farcasiu C, Andrei O-C, Grumezescu AM, Farcasiu A-T. Surface modification to modulate microbial biofilms applications in dental medicine. Materials. 2021;**14**:6994

[94] Hassan SA, Beleidy M, Alaa El-din Y. Biocompatibility and surface roughness of different sustainable dental composite blocks: Comprehensive *in vitro* study. ACS Omega. 2022;**7**:34258-34267

[95] Daguano JKMB, Milesi MTB, Rodas ACD, Weber AF, Sarkis JES, Hortellani MA, et al. In vitro biocompatibility of new bioactive lithia-silica glass-ceramics. Materials Science and Engineering: C. 2019;**94**:117-125

[96] Ille CE, Moacă E-A, Suciu M, Barbu-Tudoran L, Negruțiu M-L, Jivănescu A. The biological activity of fragmented computer-aided design/manufacturing dental materials before and after exposure to acidic environment. Medicina. 2023;**59**:104. DOI: 10.3390/medicina59010104

Chapter 3

The Impact of Hydrofluoric Acid Temperature and Application Method on the Texture of Ceramic Surfaces and the Shear Bond Strength of an Adhesive Cement

Cristiana Cuzic, Marius Octavian Pricop, Anca Jivanescu, Radu Marcel Negru, Ovidiu Stefan Cuzic, Alisia Pricop and Mihai Romînu

Abstract

All-ceramic restorations represent the fundamentals of contemporary esthetic dentistry. Adhesive dentistry has revolutionized clinical techniques for the preparation, longevity, appearance, and restoration of dental work. This study sought to assess the effects of heated hydrofluoric acid pretreatment and the influence of the application technique on the surface morphology and roughness of leucite-reinforced glass-ceramic materials. Understanding these factors is significant for comprehending the adhesive cementation process. The efficiency of the two HF application strategies and the influence of HF's temperature on the surface topography of the ceramic was observed using Scanning Electron Microscopy. On the prepared ceramic samples, resin cement was applied and light-cured in accordance with the surface conditioning techniques. The shear bond strength values were associated with the micro-retentive surface topography of the ceramic material. The SBS values between the resin cement and the ceramic material were evaluated using universal testing equipment. By utilizing digital microscopy to examine the affected surfaces of the specimens, the failure mechanisms were classified into three distinct categories: adhesive, cohesive, and mixed failure. The data was subjected to one-way and two-way analysis of variance for statistical analysis. The findings indicate that alternate treatment procedures have an impact on the surface properties of the material.

Keywords: glass-ceramic, hydrofluoric acid etching, surface treatment, adhesion, scanning electron microscopy, surface roughness, shear bond strength

1. Introduction

Dentists and other dental practitioners have been challenged with new difficulties due to recent advancements in digital dentistry. The prevalence of computer-aided design and manufacturing (CAD/CAM) technology has increased in general dentistry operations [1] due to its many advantages, such as its efficacy, user-friendliness, and therapeutic excellence. The use of this technology has unveiled several applications in the dental office and laboratory, including the production of indirect prosthodontic restorations such as inlays, veneers, crowns, fixed partial dentures, and implant abutments [2].

The advancement of CAD/CAM technology is marked by the need for durable and esthetically effective prosthodontic restorations, which may be achieved through precise and uncomplicated technical procedures [3]. Ceramic materials are widely used in the fabrication of permanent dental prostheses in contemporary dentistry. CAD/CAM systems have been developed due to their enhanced process stability, cost-effectiveness, and significant minimize of working time [4].

The principal classifications of ceramic materials include those dependent on their composition (e.g., silica-based ceramics, oxide ceramics, and resin-matrix ceramics), as well as those produced by layering, pressing, and CAD/CAM machining [5].

Under optimal conditions, clinicians may use a material that has both acceptable esthetic qualities and strong mechanical properties, capable of resisting high occlusal pressures and impervious to fracture propagation [6]. It is inherent that the microstructure of ceramics significantly influences the mechanical characteristics of the material.

Prior to bonding, it is necessary to acid-etch ceramic restorations that include a glass phase in order to achieve the desired surface structure and optimize the adhesion of resin cement [7]. It is essential to enhance resin cement adhesion. To get the maximum bond strength when utilizing adhesive-resin cement and glass ceramics, dentists may use a process that involves etching the tooth structure with 37% phosphoric acid, treating the porcelain's surface with 5–9.5% hydrofluoric acid, and using a silane coupling agent. The outcomes of the acid treatment exhibit variability since they are contingent upon the specific ceramic material being treated, the concentration of the conditioning agent, and the length of the etching process [8]. The resin exhibits a fluidic behavior and forms a strong bond inside the intricate recessed areas, hence increasing its adhesion to the etched surfaces.

After the etching process, the restoration is submerged in water and subjected to ultrasonic cleaning for a duration of five minutes. It is then dried with air and a layer of silane is applied to the intaglio surface [7]. In order to enhance the resistance to fractures of glass ceramics, it is recommended to inquire final adhesive cementation with composite resin due to their fragility and poor flexural strength [9]. Studies have shown that adhesive cementation improves fracture resistance and prolongs the longevity of the restoration [10]. When dealing with glass ceramics, it is recommended to use composite resin materials that can be polymerized using either light, dual, or chemical methods [11].

The adhesive cement's bonding strength significantly affects the retention and durability of indirect ceramic restorations. The most often used methods for studying cement types and adhesives are shear and micro tensile bond strength tests [12].

The testing technique involves analyzing the adhesion between the tooth or ceramic and the cement material to assess its capacity to withstand the stress induced by occlusal pressures. Shear bond strength values are not considered material properties since they are influenced by the substrate material and surface form, and their values vary based on the test design [13]. Prior research investigations have examined surface conditioning, the cementation process, and the expected failure of all-ceramic prosthodontic restorations at various interfaces [14]. Despite the current research on adhesive cementation methods used by dentists, recent investigations in the scientific literature suggest that the cautious application of adhesives is necessary for all-ceramic restorations. In order to decrease the incidence of clinical failure, the dentist should prioritize the dental preparation design and the expected thickness of the restoration. Previous to applying the adhesive cement, it is necessary to clean and condition the bond surfaces in order to provide strong resistance to masticatory forces and maximize durability [14].

The development and distribution of user-friendly self-etching adhesive cements by manufacturers encourage the issue of whether dentists should choose for these products instead of the traditional adhesive preparation that involves etching and priming [15].

This study aimed to investigate the impact of the application method and temperature of preheated hydrofluoric acid pretreatment on the surface morphology of leucite-reinforced glass-ceramic materials (IPS Empress CAD, Ivoclar Vivadent). Understanding this is significant for mastering the adhesive cementation process.

2. The interpretation of research data

2.1 The preparation of specimens and surface conditioning

Fifty specimens of leucite-reinforced glass-ceramic (IPS Empress, Ivoclar Vivadent, Schaan, Liechtenstein) were polished using silicon carbide papers with grit levels of #1200, #1500, and #2500 in a grinding machine (ECOMET Grinder/Polisher, Buehler). Afterward, the samples were immersed in distilled water in an ultrasonic bath for 5 minutes. An incubator (Ivoclar Vivadent Cultura) was used to warm 9.5% HF gel (Yellow Porcelain Etch, Cerkamed) for 20 minutes at 50°C.

The ceramic blocks were divided into five groups (n = 10) based on random allocation, with each group receiving a different surface treatment.

- Group 1: NT (control group)—no surface conditioning;
- Group 2: DH—a dynamic application of preheated HF-gel on the ceramic surface using continuous movements of a micro brush for 60 seconds;
- Group 3: SH—a static application of preheated HF-gel on the ceramic surface without brushing for 60 seconds;
- Group 4: DNH—a dynamic application of nonheated HF-gel (at room temperature) on the surface using active movements with a micro brush for 60 seconds;
- Group 5: SNH—a static application of nonheated HF-gel (at room temperature) on the surface without brushing for 60 seconds.

Following the HF treatment, all specimens were subjected to a 20-second cleansing using an air-water spray, followed by a 10-second session of air-drying.

2.2 Scanning electron microscopy (SEM) for surface morphology analysis

The specimens' topographic patterns were examined using a scanning electron microscope (SEM Quanta FEG 250, FEI, Hillsboro, OR, USA) and a secondary electron detector (SE). This analysis aimed to assess the impact of treatments on the surface morphology of the etched surfaces of specimens in each experimental group. The scanning electron microscope (SEM) was used in a low vacuum mode to avoid the occurrence of charge.

SEM micrographs were captured at magnifications of 1000× and 5000× to visually analyze the morphological changes on the ceramic surfaces. The objective was to detect any impacts on the ceramic area resulting from the treatments applied to the specimens. Each specimen was observed at the center of the ceramic-conditioned surface.

Figure 1(a–j) provide SEM images illustrating the notable ceramic surface morphologies of each experimental group.

Observable patterns might vary depending on the temperature and application method of hydrofluoric acid. The most suitable design for each specimen was selected for analysis. Without hydrofluoric acid (HF) treatment, the sample exhibited a consistent surface shape without noticeable ceramic microstructural characteristics.

Unlike the porous surface reported in all the analyzed etched groups, the NT group exhibited a much less retentive pattern. The study revealed that each of the HF treatments lead to significant porosities on the ceramic material's surface. After receiving surface treatments, the surface morphology of each CAD/CAM block underwent substantial alterations. The alterations in surface roughness were readily discernible on the SEM micrographs.

The microscopic examination demonstrates that the ceramic conditioning procedure has an impact on the surface micro retentions of ceramics.

2.3 Assessment of surface roughness

The surface roughness was evaluated using a contact profilometer (Surftest SJ-201, Mitutoyo, Kanagawa, Japan). Prior to completing measurements, the profilometer was calibrated using a reference sample given by the manufacturer.

Two perpendicular measurements were obtained along certain orientations after surface conditioning, starting from the center point of each sample (with a cutoff length of 0.25 mm).

The analysis documented the Ra values, which indicate the average roughness of the treated surfaces. These values are calculated by measuring the absolute roughness of the peaks and valleys from a reference plane. The measurements were denoted in micrometers (μm) and the average of the measurements was recorded.

Ten roughness measures were conducted for each group, and the results are shown in **Table 1**.

2.4 Shear bond tests are conducted to evaluate the strength of adhesive bonds

All specimens were treated with a silane coupling agent (Clearfil Ceramic Primer Plus; Kuraray Noritake Dental Inc., Tokyo, Japan) following instructions provided by the manufacturer.

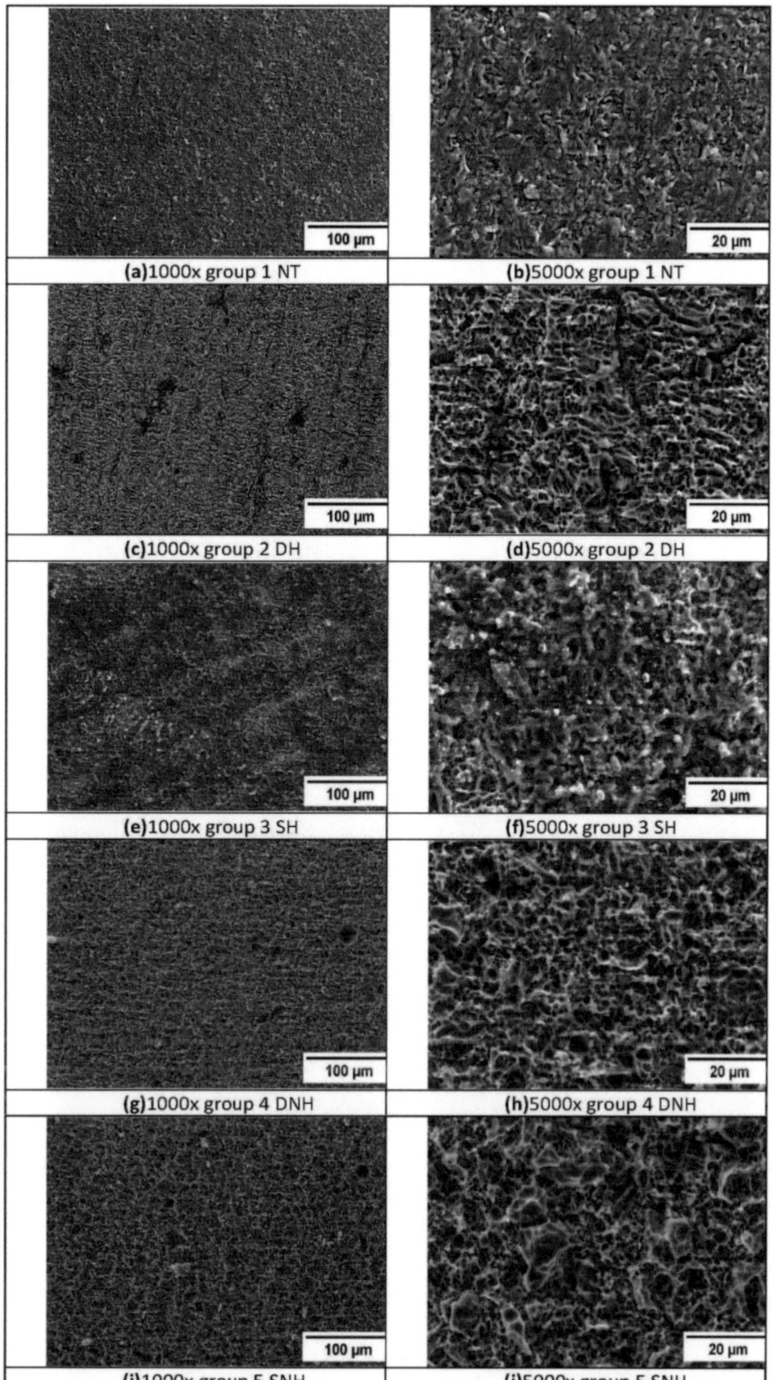

Figure 1.
(a–j) SEM evaluation images with significant ceramic surface morphologies of all experimental groups. (a) 1000× group 1 NT, (b) 5000× group 1 NT, (c) 1000× group 2 DH, (d) 5000× group 2 DH, (e) 1000× group 3 SH, (f) 5000× group 3 SH, (g) 1000× group 4 DNH, (h) 5000× group 4 DNH, (i) 1000× group 5 SNH, (j) 5000× group 5 SNH.

Roughness $R_a\,(\mu m)$					
Group specimen	**NT**	**DH**	**SH**	**DNH**	**SNH**
1	0.27	0.56	0.87	1.05	1.02
2	0.25	0.51	0.83	0.85	1.18
3	0.26	0.52	0.78	0.86	0.99
4	0.24	0.62	0.75	0.94	0.87
5	0.27	0.56	0.87	0.91	0.95
6	0.28	0.72	0.77	1.02	0.88
7	0.30	0.64	0.91	0.98	1.16
8	0.29	0.61	0.92	0.96	1.07
9	0.27	0.74	0.94	0.84	1.22
10	0.30	0.47	0.82	0.93	1.23
Mean	0.273	0.595	0.846	0.934	1057
SD	0.020	0.088	0.067	0.071	0.128

Table 1.
The roughness measurements results. Mean—average value, SD—standard deviation.

Precisely designed, translucent cylindrical items with parallel ends were methodically shaped out from a polyvinyl tube that had an inner diameter of 3 mm and a height of 5 mm. For each specimen, a single cylinder was used to adhere the adhesive cement to the prepared surfaces. Once placed on the surface of the treated samples, each cylindrical support made of polyvinyl was carefully filled with cement (Panavia V5, Kuraray Noritake Dental Inc., Tokyo, Japan). Subsequently, adhesive cement cylinders were distributed onto the treated surfaces and subjected to light-curing for a duration of 20 seconds utilizing a DTE LUX-E Plus Curing Light (Woodpecker, 1000 mW/cm^2) LED curing device. The LED curing device was activated in contact with the tube due to its 1 mm thickness. The polyvinyl tubes were removed after the adhesive got fully cured. Before conducting the bond strength tests, all specimens were immersed in distilled water for a period of 7 days.

Requirements for conducting shear tests:

The Zwick/Roell Z005 universal machine was used to conduct the testing, possessing the following technical specifications:

- the Zwick/Roell Z005 universal machine is equipped with a force cell of 5 (kN) in uniaxial stress, in the accuracy class 0.5 on the force measurement range 1–130 (%) according to ISO 7500-1;

- the Zwick/Roell Z005 machine owns the TestXpert data processing software and an incremental extensometer with a maximum error of ±1 (μm) for the differential measurement of the displacement between two measuring points in the range of 20–200 (μm) (class of precision 0.5).

The machine is prepared with equipment for conducting tensile, compression, and three-point bending tests.

The tests were carried out in controlled movement mode, at an ambient temperature of 23°C, as follows:

- pre-load at 2 (N), with a traverse speed of 2 (mm/min);
- shear test with a crossbar travel speed of 0.5 (mm/min);
- real-time recording of the force F and the displacement of the crossbar.

The specimens were fixed using a precision vice, and the tester blade was positioned perpendicular to the adhesive cement cylinder at a 90° angle. The specimens underwent shear loading along the interface until complete failure, which was indicated by the highest recorded force F_max. The force was measured using the TestXpert II software [16].

The shear strength τ_{max}, expressed in MPa, was determined from the conventional formula (1):

$$\tau_{max} = F_{max} / A. \tag{1}$$

Before performing the tests, the diameter of the specimens was measured using a caliper with an accuracy of 0.01 (mm), in three different directions.

F_{max} represents the maximum force recorded at failure, expressed in newton (N), and A the shear area, i.e., the area of a circle having diameter d, expressed in (mm^2) from the formula (2):

$$A = \pi \cdot d^2 / 4 \tag{2}$$

Figure 2(a–e) show the force-displacement curves for each treatment type, with three curves per group, selected randomly.

2.5 Statistical analysis

The data were subjected to statistical analysis using SPSS Statistics 29.0 software (IBM, New York, USA, 2022) at a significance level of $\alpha = 0.05$.

The SBS data underwent preliminary testing for normality and homogeneity using the Shapiro-Wilk and Levene tests. The initial null hypothesis, asserting that the variable SBS follows a normal distribution, was not found to be statistically significant. The second null hypothesis posits that the variances of the five groups are the same, hence lacking statistical significance in their differences.

In addition, a one-way analysis of variance (ANOVA) and the post hoc Tukey HSD test were used to see whether there were any significant differences in terms of SBS across the five groups. The null hypothesis of equal mean SBS levels across all five groups was rejected.

A two-way analysis of variance (ANOVA) using a general linear model was conducted to investigate the differential impact of temperature (heated or non-heated HF-gel) and application regime (static or dynamic application) on the dependent variable SBS. The groups DH, SH, DNH, and SNH were included in the analysis [16].

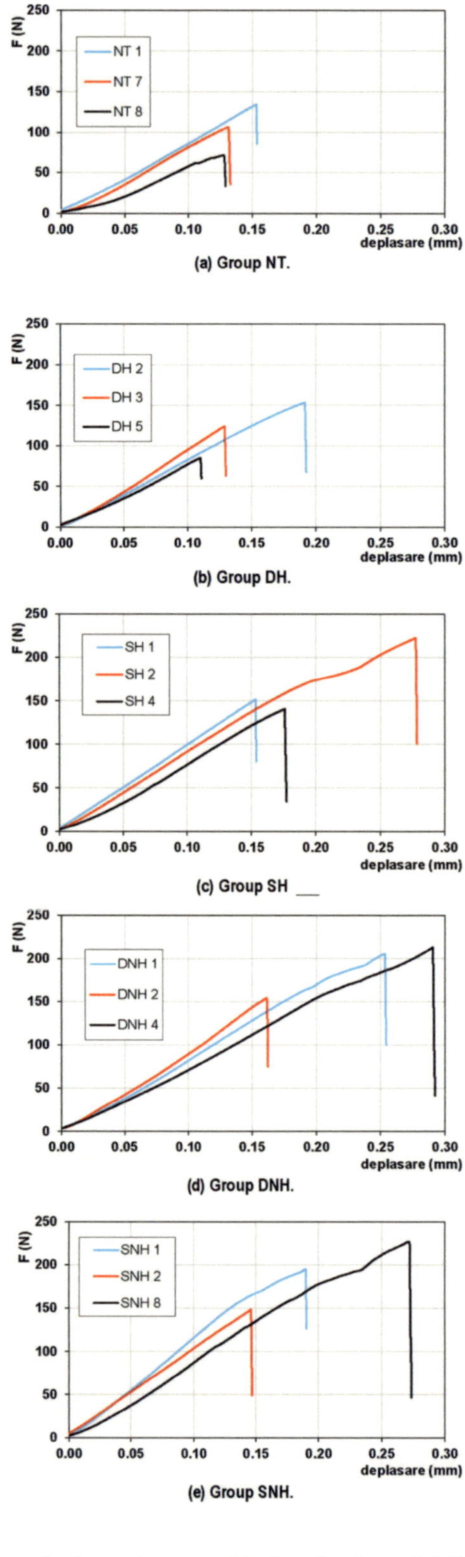

Figure 2

(a–e). *Force-displacement curves for the specimens tested in shear bond tests. (a) Group NT. (b) Group DH. (c) Group SH. (d) Group DNH. (e) Group SNH.*

2.6 Digital microscopy for fracture surfaces

The failure mechanisms of the ceramic and adhesive cement interfaces were analyzed at a 50× magnification using a digital microscope installed at the CMDTCA (Research Centre in Dental Medicine Using Conventional and Alternative Technologies) at the university research center. The failure types were categorized as shown in **Figure 3(a** and **b)** into three distinct groups: adhesive (A), which refers to failure occurring at the bond surfaces between the ceramic and the resin cement substrate; cohesive (C), which refers to failure of either the ceramic or the adhesive cement substrate; and mixed (M), which combines both adhesive and cohesive failures [16].

The use of static surface treatment procedures enhanced the adhesive strength between the ceramic material and resin cement. The SBS was significantly affected by two contributing factors: the temperature of the hydrofluoric acid (whether heated or not) and the application method (static or dynamic). The temperature at which HF is delivered has a significant impact compared to the technique of application.

The final findings are not statistically substantially affected by the interaction between these two factors in terms of SBS shear strength.

There is no statistically significant variation in the mean SBS values across the NT, DH, and SH preparations. The surface treatments applied to the DNH and SNH groups resulted in average SBS values that were 56.32% and 74.88% higher, respectively, compared to the NT control group. The SBS values for DNH and SNH conditioning increased by 65% and 84.59%, respectively, compared to the DH group, indicating the impact of these two parameters. The preparations of the SH and DNH groups do not exhibit statistically significant results in terms of SBS shear strength due to the conflicting effects of the two influencing factors. However, the SNH group shows a notable 35.73% enhancement in SBS compared to the SH group. The only

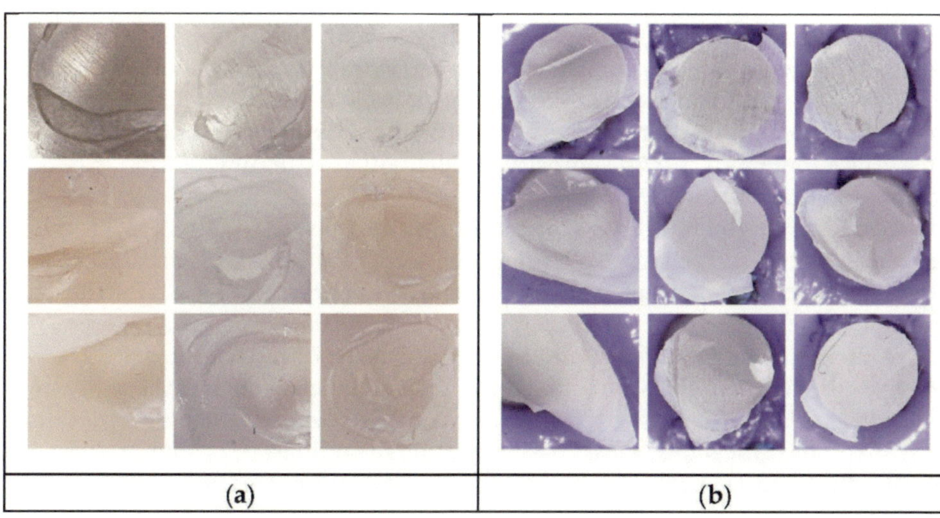

Figure 3.
(a and b) Images showing the typical fractographic characteristics after the impact of the shear test: (a) ceramic interfaces after SBS forces; (b) resin cement interfaces after SBS tests. Adhesive (failure at the bond interfaces where the ceramic and the resin cement substrate were connected), cohesive (failure of at least one of the substrates—the ceramic or the composite resin), and mixed failures can be observed.

difference in the shear strengths of the DNH and SNH groups is in the manner in which HF was applied, and this discrepancy is deemed negligible [16].

Resin cement is essential for ensuring the long-term effectiveness of ceramic-based dental restorations. A fracture in the restorative material or inadequate adherence at the cement contact might cause the restoration to fail [17]. The intaglio surfaces of all ceramic restorations have been specifically roughened by etching. This roughening process is said to enhance the surface area, allowing for better adhesion between the ceramic surface and resin-based components [18].

Acid selectively dissolves the crystalline or amorphous phases of the ceramic, resulting in unsaturated oxygen connections that may interact with phosphate monomers with dual capacities [19]. Hydrofluoric acid creates porous and uneven surfaces, as well as micro retention sites, in ceramic materials by precisely eliminating the glassy or crystalline matrix. The microporous ceramic surfaces undergo expansion, hence increasing their surface area and facilitating resin infiltration [20].

Chemical conditioning, such as acid etching, improves the roughness and energy of the ceramic surface. This process increases micromechanical retention and the ability of the primer to adhere, leading to higher bond strength [21]. The primary factors influencing bond strength values are the surface energy of the material and the interfacial tension between the material itself and the adhesive [22]. Previous literature studies show how while there is no direct relationship between surface roughness and surface energy, an increase in surface energy leads to higher bond strength values [23]. The use of HF treatment and silanization resulted in the highest bond strength values for feldspathic ceramic [24]. The most effective surface treatment for leucite-based ceramics is etching by using a combination of hydrofluoric acid and silane [25].

With the introduction of glass-based ceramics and a greater understanding of the benefits of adhesive cementation in dentistry, hydrofluoric acid has become a common surface conditioner for restorative materials [26]. Universal adhesives facilitate clinical application processes for practitioners while strengthening them [27].

Though a specific silane treatment is necessary, particularly for feldspathic ceramics, previous studies have shown that the primary factor for achieving a strong bond is the mechanical interlocking that occurs due to the roughness of the ceramic surface [28]. Roughness is a major surface property of restorative materials that affect the ability of abrasive and mechanically organized substances to interact with their external environment. Material adhesion is influenced by other parameters apart from surface roughness, such as porosity, residual microstructural tension, composition, and internal defects [29].

The bond strength between two materials may be assessed in vitro using tensile, microshear, and shear techniques. The basic concept of these tests is to subject the specimen to stresses that exert stress on the adhesive contact until the failure of the specimen becomes apparent. Each of these tests has both benefits and drawbacks, although none is universally acknowledged as the optimal approach [30]. Furthermore, the results may be influenced by several factors such as the shape of the specimen, the brittleness of the substrate, and the speed at which the cross-head moves [31]. The critical load measured during the shear bond tests did not accurately represent the bond strengths attained by the various surface treatments at the adhesive interface.

Shorter processing times, fewer costs, and better patient results have resulted from the development of CAD/CAM technology. Moreover, digital dental technology enables the use of same-day restorations for patients, hence eliminating the need for many sessions and interim restorations. Consequently, novel ceramic materials have been developed explicitly for use with CAD/CAM systems. The purpose of developing these biomaterials was to meet the specific demands of dental restorations, such as the need for strength, durability, and biocompatibility. In general, the use of CAD/CAM technology in dentistry has substantially improved the quality of treatment that dentists can deliver to their patients, while also streamlining processes in laboratories and clinics.

The limitations of the SBS test in imitating clinical loading forces and aging within the oral environment should be noted as they may have an influence on this in vitro investigation. It is certainly suggested to conduct additional research to investigate the effects of ceramic surface conditioning on bond strengths in a clinical setting, focusing on the most optimal methods of ceramic surface conditioning.

The success of the prosthodontic treatment relies significantly on the dentist's capacity to choose the appropriate restoration material, manufacturing process, and cementation or bonding processes, taking into account both the circumstances within the oral cavity and the esthetic goal. The clinical efficacy of dental restorations' cementation procedures will be influenced by the surface conditioning and its continuous enhancement [16].

3. Conclusions

The limitations of this study permit the following conclusion to be drawn:

1. Both the temperature of the HF and the technique of its application significantly affect SBS values, although the temperature has a more pronounced influence. The shear bond strength values show an increase in comparison to the control group when subjected to the other four types of ceramic treatment.

2. The ceramic surface patterns are determined by the application technique and temperature of hydrofluoric acid.

3. Following the removal of the bond, the interfaces were inspected, revealing the presence of all three types of bonding failures: adhesive, cohesive, and mixed. The occurrence of cohesive failure was limited to the ceramic material, whereas no cohesive fracture was seen in the adhesive cement.

Conflict of interest

The authors declare no conflict of interest.

Author details

Cristiana Cuzic[1,2*], Marius Octavian Pricop[3,4], Anca Jivanescu[1,2], Radu Marcel Negru[4,5], Ovidiu Stefan Cuzic[6], Alisia Pricop[7] and Mihai Romînu[4,8]

1 Faculty of Dental Medicine, Department of Prosthodontics, University of Medicine and Pharmacy "Victor Babes", Timisoara, Romania

2 Research Center of Digital and Advanced Technique for Endodontic, Restorative and Prosthetic Treatment (TADERP), Timisoara, Romania

3 Faculty of Dentistry, Department of Oral and Maxillofacial Surgery, University of Medicine and Pharmacy "Victor Babes", Timisoara, Romania

4 Research Center in Dental Medicine Using Conventional and Alternative Technologies, School of Dental Medicine, University of Medicine and Pharmacy "Victor Babes", Timisoara, Romania

5 Department of Mechanics and Strength of Materials, Politehnica University, Romania

6 Department of Hydrotechnical Engineering, Polytechnica University, Romania

7 Faculty of Dental Medicine, University of Medicine and Pharmacy "Victor Babes", Romania

8 Faculty of Dentistry, Department of Prosthesis Technology and Dental Materials, University of Medicine and Pharmacy "Victor Babes", Timisoara, Romania

*Address all correspondence to: pricop.cristiana@umft.ro

References

[1] Blatz MB, Conejo J. The current state of chairside digital dentistry and materials. Dental Clinics of North America. 2019;**63**(2):175-197

[2] Papadopoulos C, Dionysopoulos D, Tolidis K, Kouros P, Koliniotou-Koumpia E, Tsitrou EA. Structural integrity evaluation of large MOD restorations fabricated with a bulk-fill and a CAD/CAM resin composite material. Operative Dentistry. 2019;**44**(3):312-332

[3] Kömürcüoğlu MB, Sağırkaya E, Tulga A. Influence of different surface treatments on bond strength of novel CAD/CAM re-storative materials to resin cement. Journal of Advanced Prosthodontics. 2017;**9**(6):439-446

[4] Miyazaki T, Miyazaki T, Hotta Y, Kunii J, Kuriyama S, Tamaki Y. A review of dental CAD/CAM: Current status and future perspectives from 20 years of experience. Dental Materials Journal. 2009;**28**(1):44-56

[5] Gracis S, Thompson VP, Ferencz JL, Silva NRFA, Bonfante EA. A new classification system for all-ceramic and ceramic-like restorative materials. The International Journal of Prosthodontics. 2015;**28**(3):227-235

[6] Zhang Y, Kelly JR. Dental ceramics for restoration and metal veneering. Dental Clinics of North America. 2017;**61**(4):797-819

[7] Bajraktarova-Valjakova E, Grozdanov A, Guguvcevski L, et al. Acid etching as surface treatment method for luting of glass-ceramic restorations, part 1: Acids, application protocol and etching effectiveness. Macedonian Journal of Medical Sciences. 2018;**6**(3):568-573

[8] Grégoire G, Poulet P-P, Sharrock P, et al. Hydrofluoric acid etching versus self-etching glass ceramic primer: Consequences on the interface with resin cements. Oral Health Care. 2019;**4**:1-7

[9] Bindl A, Richter B, Mörmann WH. Survival of ceramic computer-aided design/manufactoring crowns bonded to preparations with reduced macroretention geometry. International Journal of Prosthodontics. 2005;**18**:219-224

[10] Attia A, Abdelaziz KM, Freitag S, Kern M. Fracture load composite resin and feldspatic all-ceramic CAD/CAM crowns. The Journal of Prosthetic Dentistry. 2006;**95**:117-123

[11] Conrad HJ, Seong W-J, Pesun IJ. Current ceramic materials and systems with clinical recommandations: A systematic review. The Journal of Prosthetic Dentistry. 2007;**98**:389-404

[12] De Munck J, van Landuyt K, Peumans M, et al. A critical review of the durability of adhesion to tooth tissue: Methods and results. Journal of Dental Research. 2005;**84**(2):118-132

[13] Van Noort R, Noroozi S, Howard IC, Cardew G. A critique of bond strength measurements. Journal of Dentistry. 1989;**17**(2):61-67

[14] Cuzic C, Pricop MO, Jivanescu A, Ursoniu S, Negru RM, Rominu M. Assessment of different techniques for adhesive cementation of all-ceramic systems. Medicina. 2022;**58**:1006

[15] Rohr N, Fischer J. Tooth surface treatment strategies for adhesive cementation. Journal of Advanced Prosthodontics. 2017;**9**:85-92

[16] Cuzic C, Jivanescu A, Negru RM, Hulka I, Rominu M. The influence of hydrofluoric acid temperature and application technique on ceramic surface texture and shear bond strength of an adhesive cement. Materials. 2023;**16**(12):4303

[17] Qeblawi DM, Muñoz CA, Brewer JD, Monaco EA Jr. The effect of zirconia surface treatment on flexural strength and shear bond strength to a resin cement. The Journal of Prosthetic Dentistry. 2010;**103**(4):210-220

[18] Carrabba M, Vichi A, Louca C, Ferrari M. Comparison of traditional and simplified methods for repairing CAD/CAM feldspathic ceramics. Journal of Advanced Prosthodontics. 2017;**9**(4):257-264

[19] Yen TW, Blackman RB, Baez RJ. Effect of acid etching on the flexural strength of a feldspathic porcelain and a castable glass ceramic. The Journal of Prosthetic Dentistry. 1993;**70**(3):224-233

[20] Timokhin AR, Komarova L. Chemical reaction of ammonium bifluoride with quartz glass. Glass and Ceramics. 1985;**42**:267-269

[21] Sturz CR, Faber F-J, Scheer M, et al. Effects of various chair-side surface treatment methods on dental restorative materials with respect to contact angles and surface roughness. Dental Materials Journal. 2015;**34**(6):796-813

[22] Della-Bona A. Characterizing ceramics and the interfacial adhesion to resin: II—The relationship of surface treatment, bond strength, interfacial toughness and fractography. Journal of Applied Oral Science. 2005;**13**(2):101-109

[23] Lung CYK, Matinlinna JP. Aspects of silane coupling agents and surface conditioning in dentistry: An overview. Dental Materials. 2012;**28**(5):467-477

[24] Özcan M. Adhesion to zirconia used for dental restorations: A systematic review and meta-analysis. The Journal of Adhesive Dentistry. 2015;**17**(1):7-26

[25] Özcan M, Bernasconi M. Repair bond strength of microhybrid, nanohybrid and nanofilled resin composites: Effect of substrate resin type, surface conditioning and ageing. Clinical Oral Investigations. 2013;**17**(7):1751-1758

[26] Zaghloul H, Elkassas DW, Haridy MF. Effect of incorporation of silane in the bonding agent on the repair potential of machinable esthetic blocks. European Journal of Dental. 2014;**8**(1):44-52

[27] Wahsh MM, Ghallab OH. Influence of different surface treatments on micro shear bond strength of repair resin composite to two CAD/CAM esthetic restorative materials. Tanta Dental Journal. 2015;**12**:178-184

[28] de Melo RM, Valandro LF, Bottino MA. Microtensile bond strength of a repair composite to leucite-reinforced feldspathic ceramic. Brazilian Dental Journal. 2007;**18**(4):314-319

[29] Kelly JR, Nishimura I, Campbell SD. Ceramics in dentistry: Historical roots and current perspectives. The Journal of Prosthetic Dentistry. 1996;**75**(1):18-32

[30] Sadek FT, Cury AH, Monticelli F, et al. The influence of the cutting speed on bond strength and integrity of microtensile specimens. Dental Materials. 2005;**21**(12):1144-1149

[31] Goracci C, Sadek FT, Monticelli F, et al. Influence of substrate, shape, and thickness on microtensile specimens' structural integrity and their measured bond strengths. Dental Materials. 2004;**20**(7):643-654

Chapter 4

Prosthetic Management of Tooth Malposition

Yosra Gassara, Rim Kallala, Emna Boudabous, Ines Azouzi and Zohra Nouira

Abstract

Tooth malposition can negatively affect the appearance of a person's smile. In these cases, it is essential to conduct a comprehensive clinical and radiological examination to determine the type and extent of the tooth malposition before selecting the appropriate treatment option. Orthodontic treatment is generally used to correct mild to severe malocclusions. In cases where the tooth malposition is associated with other dental issues such as tooth discoloration, ceramic restorations may be a suitable alternative.

Keywords: dental veneers, dental crowns, dental bridges, tooth malposition, malocclusion

1. Introduction

Tooth malposition may impair the esthetic smile. In these cases, it is essential to conduct a comprehensive clinical and radiological examination to determine the type and extent of the tooth malposition before selecting the appropriate treatment option.

After cephalometric analysis, orthodontic treatment, with or without orthognathic surgery is considered to be the conventional approach for correcting mild to severe malocclusions. The orthodontic treatment has several disadvantages. First, according to Fink DF, the duration of an orthodontic treatment is from 19.4 to 27.9 months [1]. This long period does not encourage patients for the surgical- orthodontic correction. Second, relapse after orthodontic treatment is frequent, it has been attributed to tongue posture, treatment parameters, growth pattern, and surgical fragment instability. In addition to that, linked to orthodontic intervention, numerous local effects with manifestation on dento-maxillary structures are described, as enamel demineralization and discoloration, root resorption, and gingivitis [2].

All of these factors lead patients to find another treatment modality and have inspired clinicians to opt for ceramic prosthesis to correct malocclusion. This restorative approach is commonly referred to as "Instant Orthodontics" or "Two appointment orthodontics" [2, 3].

Prosthetic management of tooth malposition involves the use of dental prostheses, such as dental bridges, crowns, and veneers, to correct the appearance and function of misaligned teeth. The treatment approach will depend on the severity and cause of the tooth malposition.

For mild to moderate cases of tooth malposition, dental veneers can be used to improve the appearance of the affected teeth. Veneers are thin, custom-made shells that are placed over the front surface of the teeth to conceal any cosmetic imperfections, such as tooth discoloration, cracks, or minor misalignments.

For more severe cases, dental crowns or bridges may be necessary. Dental crowns are used to cover damaged or discolored teeth, while dental bridges can replace missing teeth. The prostheses can be designed to correct the alignment of the teeth, which can improve the overall appearance and function of the patient's mouth [3].

Orthodontic treatment may also be necessary to correct severe tooth malposition, and the use of dental prostheses may be combined with orthodontic treatment to achieve optimal results.

The practitioner should evaluate the position of teeth and gum, discuss the various available treatment, and recommend to the patient the best option to achieve an esthetic outcome [4].

This chapter aims to describe different types of teeth malposition: Misalignments, open bite, crossbite, and deep bite. We include a discussion of preparation and possible prosthetic solutions for the correction of mispositioned anterior teeth.

2. Ethical concerns regarding restorative correction of mispositioned teeth

The correction of mispositioned teeth using fixed prosthesis presents significant clinical as well as ethical quandaries. According to the American Dental Association Principles of Ethics and Code of Professional Conduct, the clinician should respect some principles when treating misaligned teeth restoratively.

Five fundamental principles form the foundation of the American Dental Association Code: patient autonomy, non-maleficence, beneficence, justice, and veracity.

Respecting these principles, the dentist should choose the more conservative method following the "therapeutic gradient" (**Figure 1**) and exhibit the pros and cons of every possible treatment approach.

The decision to restore an anterior tooth with crown or veneer depends on some criteria. These criteria should be considered when evaluating a patient for esthetic rehabilitation: thorough medical and dental histories, clinical photographs, study casts, periapical and panoramic radiographs, the diagnostic wax-up/mock-up, as well as, the use of a planning technique like the digital smile design (DSD).

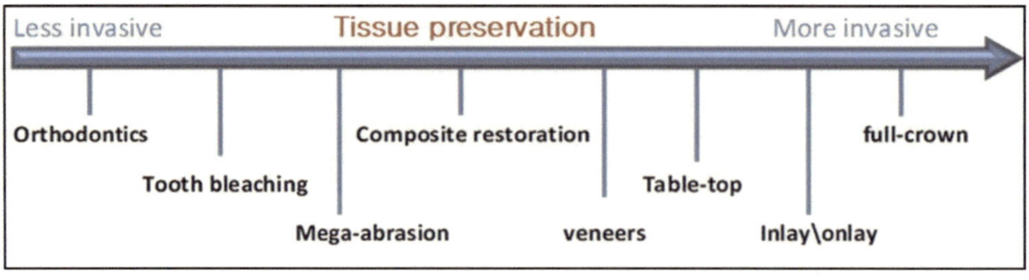

Figure 1.
Therapeutic gradient for tooth malposition.

3. Clinical examination

A comprehensive evaluation of the patient before initiation of any esthetic rehabilitation is important to establish a treatment plan. For the long-term success of any treatment, a detailed analysis of the patient involving medical/dental history and clinical examination includes assessment of oral soft tissues and dental hard tissues [5]:

- Pernicious habits
- Hereditary syndromes which feature hypoparathyroidism
- Dietary habits
- Present and future restorative and oral care
- Previous dental visits and treatments, past dental problems, previous conditions, and patient responses to procedures

After the entire medical and dental history is complete, extraoral examination is performed involving:

- Facial contours
- Facial symmetry
- Lip position at rest and smile
- Midline axis
- Temporomandibular joint
- Muscle tension
- Mastication

After that, a detailed clinical evaluation of all determinants of the mouth such as periodontal condition, dental hard tissues, oral soft tissue, occlusion, and esthetic analysis is done.

Anterior restoration must be esthetically pleasing for patients, functional, and biocompatible with the soft tissue.

Following points should be evaluated in esthetic rehabilitation [6–9]:

- Gingival levels
- Gingival embrasure
- Gingival recession
- Periodontal pockets

- Plaque and calculus
- Mobility of a tooth
- Tooth-tooth relationship
- Tooth-gingival relationship
- Caries lesions
- Defective restorations
- Tooth defects such as erosion, abrasion, and attrition.
- Overjet
- Overbite
- Amount and localization of the diastema
- Maxillary and mandibular relationship
- The midline
- Smile line
- Shape, size, and color of teeth
- Relationship of teeth with the lips and face of the patients on the esthetic reconstruction area.

4. Esthetic planning project

4.1 Wax mock-up

Prosthodontic treatment aims to use a minimally invasive approach to improve the appearance of the smile.

The wax-up\ mock-up binomial is a guide for restorative dentists and for laboratory technicians to get the best esthetic, phonetic, and functional outcome with preservation of maximum dental tissue [10].

The diagnostic cast should be waxed referring to the important elements for an esthetic smile design: tooth dimension, axial inclination, gingival level, teeth alignment, tooth-tooth relationship, embrasures and gingival architecture [11].

In addition to that, a color-coded wax-up (**Figure 2**) can be used for easy identification of zones that need reduction and areas that require addition of materials. This color code facilitates the quantification of removed dental tissue or of the thickness of ceramic to be added. If they are minimal, porcelain laminate veneers must be the first option when planning for an indirect restoration for the esthetic sector. According to Jacopo Castelnuovo, [12] to enhance and standardize the predictability of such

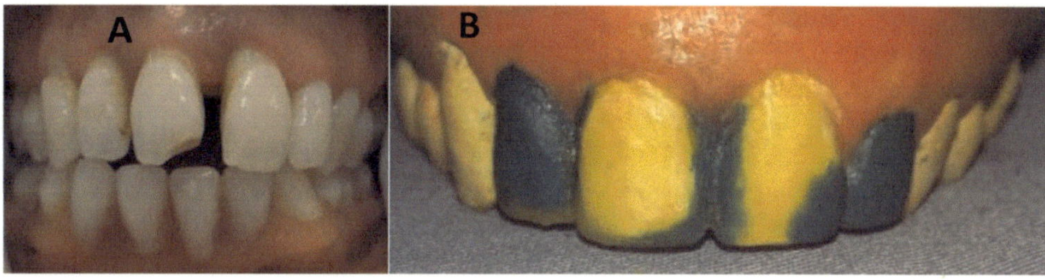

Figure 2.
Color-coded wax-up.

restorations, a minimum 50% of tooth preparation should be in enamel. Therefore, before starting the preparation, the practitioner can make the right decision with a color-coded wax-up.

A: Initial case, B: The yellow wax corresponds to areas which necessitate dental tissue removal, green areas correspond to the additional thickness needed in this situation: interface between silicone matrix and wax showing the amount of removal.

The wax-up should be tried in the patient's mouth with a resin mock-up in order to validate the prosthetic project.

4.2 Esthetic virtual planning project

To achieve esthetic and functional harmony, the prosthesis should be similar to the mock-up. The adaptation of the prosthesis, shape, size, and color of the new elements in relation with the soft tissue and the whole face are very important in the decision-making.

A large number of errors can occur at the various stages of the traditional prosthetic treatment. Each stage requires a transfer of two-dimensional and three-dimensional (3D) data between operators [13].

Thus, contemporary digital technologies may provide advantageous features to help in this diagnostic treatment step, assisting clinician in visualizing and measuring dentogingival discrepancies, as well as allowing patients to previsualize the therapy planning.

DSD is based on a clear extraoral and intraoral photographic protocol, which is necessary for the esthetic analysis of some specific elements [14]:

- Facial analysis.
- Dentofacial analysis.
- Dentolabial analysis (incisal edge position, smile line, buccal corridor).
- Dentogingival analysis.
- Dental analysis (inter- and intra-tooth relationships).

All data are arranged in a slideshow by means of general presentation software (Keynote for Apple users; PowerPoint for PC users) or dedicated software (e.g. Digital Smile System, DSS) that allow a digital previsualization of the final smile.

In addition to that, DSD may aid to making decision between restoring anterior teeth with porcelain veneers or all-ceramic crowns. In situations of tooth malposition, DSD helps us to quantify the amount of the modifications needed on every single tooth to obtain an anterior sector in harmony with the patient's dentition. [14]

This approach allows to measure the residual enamel tissue after tooth preparation, if an important quantity is eliminated and the dentin is exposed, bonding will be compromised and porcelain veneers will not be indicated.

Today with the evolution of software and digital dentistry, the esthetic virtual planning project is essential before starting any prosthetic treatment.

This project is made by using patient photographs and basic image processing software to carry out the analysis and propose ideal and appropriate esthetic designs in the form of a virtual wax-up with precise shapes and measurements that can be transcribed into a physical wax-up.

Thanks to the validated virtual planning, a model of the future project will then be produced in order to materialize the final treatment before any irreversible gesture. It will be a key communication tool between the patient and the various treatment stakeholders.

Some software like Exocad smile creator make it possible to create a virtual wax-up using the optical impression of the dental arches with more possibilities of individualization to finally obtain a 3D design of the virtual project. This virtual wax-up can help the practitioner to choose the appropriate prosthetic decision by evaluating the amount of dental tissue to be removed. If this quantity is minimal, the malposition can be corrected by veneers. If the preparation will be important, the indication of full coverage crowns will be necessary.

5. Misalignments \ crowding or dental malposition

Malocclusions are often caused by multiple misaligned teeth due to rotation, labial and lingual tipping [15–17]. The evaluation of the level of malocclusion is mainly subjective and so it may be assessed as minor, mild, moderate, or severe [2]. Many classifications of teeth crowding have been reported in the literature such as the malalignment Index of Van Kirk and Pennel (1959) which presents three scores: 0, 1, and 2 depending on the grading of the tooth displacement and rotation [15].

Score 0: Ideal alignment: absence of any apparent deviation from the ideal arch line (**Figure 3**).

Score 1: Minor malalignment that includes two types:

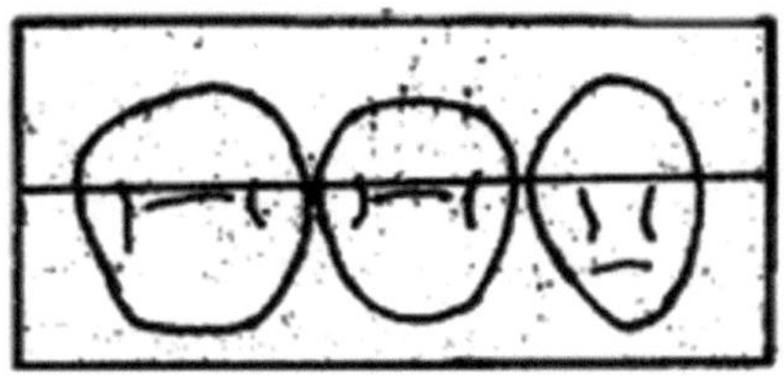

Figure 3.
Ideal alignment.

- Minor malalignment due to rotation: the angle between the line projected through the contact areas of misaligned tooth and the ideal alignment is less than 45° (**Figure 4**).
- Minor malalignment due to displacement: both contact areas of misaligned tooth are moved less than 1.5 mm in the same direction from their ideal position (**Figure 5**).

Score 2: Major malalignment that includes two types:

- Major malalignment due to rotation: the angle between the line projected through the contact areas of misaligned tooth and the ideal alignment is 45° or larger (**Figure 6**).
- Major malalignment due to displacement: both contact areas of misaligned tooth are moved by 1.5 mm or more from their ideal position (**Figure 7**).

Distinguishing between minor and major misalignments can be made using wax casts. So, the correct alignment of the incisal margins will be waxed up, and the ideal placement of the anterior teeth will be identified [16]. Due to the length of treatment

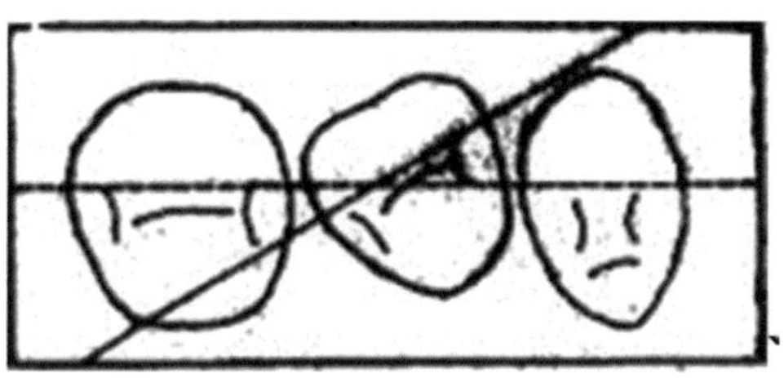

Figure 4.
Rotation: Less than 45 degrees.

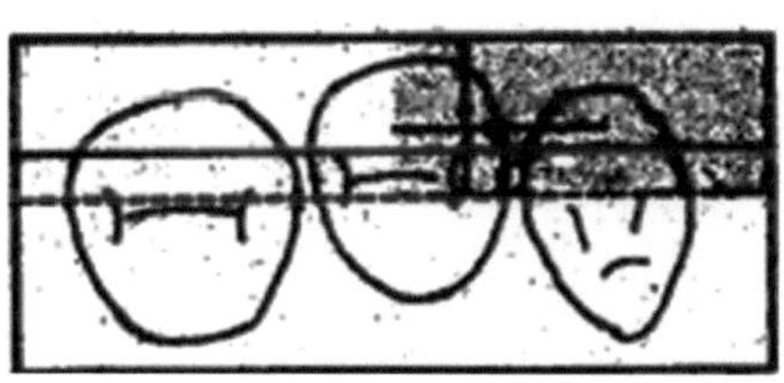

Figure 5.
Displacement: Less than 1.5 millimeters.

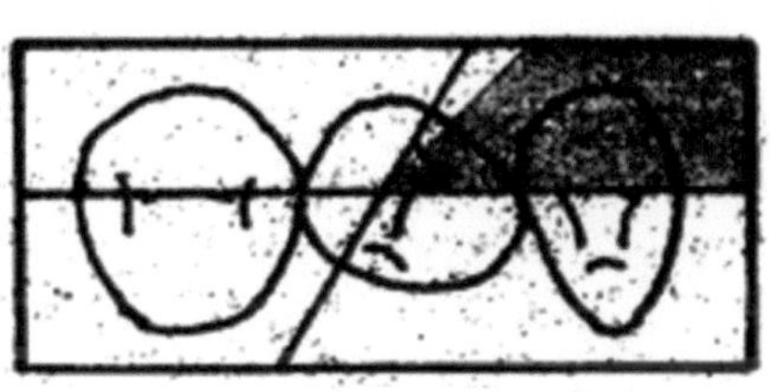

Figure 6.
Rotation: More than 45 degrees.

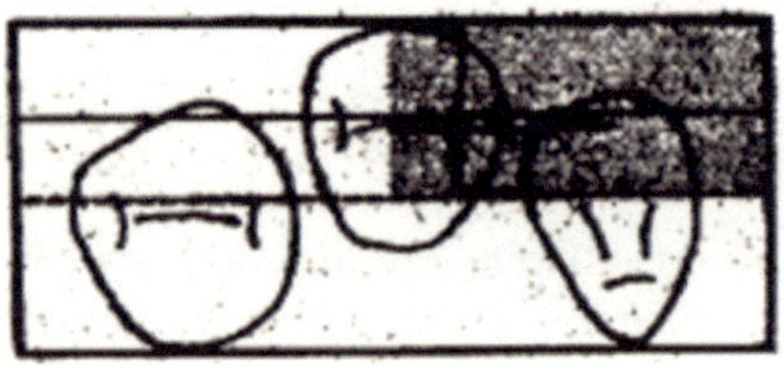

Figure 7.
Displacement: More than 1.5 millimeters.

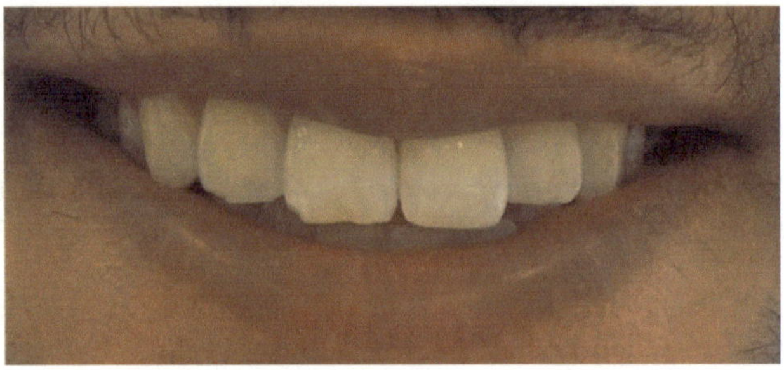

Figure 8.
Minor malalignment.

duration and the high perceived costs of transparent aligners and orthodontic therapy, using porcelain veneers to correct minor misalignment issues (**Figure 8**) can be an optimal choice.

Additionally, if the incisors are positioned lingually to the arch, it may only be necessary to slightly reduce their incisal edges in order to create a new point of contact for the porcelain veneers to correct crowding incisors. So, no-preparation porcelain veneers are more readily accepted by patients, particularly those having dental phobia or objecting to have their tooth structure removed [18].

When opting for porcelain veneers, removed tooth structure's amount will be diminished. Preservation of the enamel tissue is crucial when reconstructing teeth with porcelain veneers for a number of reasons including the elastic modulus of the enamel, which is stiffer than that of feldspathic ceramic and prevents ceramic fracture by absorbing stress. Additionally, the shear bond strength has become more significant and bonding predictability and success have enhanced when there was more present enamel [12].

Consequently, restoring an esthetic smile with ceramic crowns in cases of severe misalignment may result in the creation of teeth with pleasing inherent proportions to one another as well as a pleasant tooth arrangement that is in harmony with the patient's gingiva, lips, and face [19].

Full crowns are more appropriate when crowding of the teeth is accompanied by other anomalies such dental anomalies of structure, form, or color (**Figure 9**).

6. Open bite

In order to ensure long-term stability, a rigorous diagnosis is necessary for anterior open bite (AOB) which is a vertical malocclusion of the anterior teeth occurring when the posterior teeth are in occlusion. Some authors claim that the term

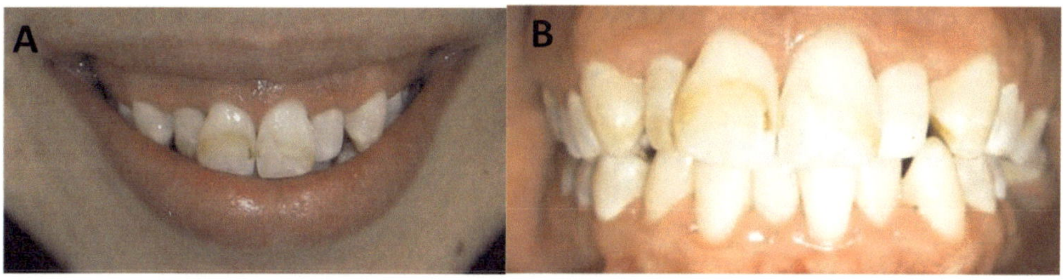

Figure 9.
Teeth crowding associated with fluorosis. A: Patient's smile, B: Front view.

"open bite" can refer to incisal end-to-end contact as well as situations where there is no incisive contact. The anterior open bite is influenced by a number of factors, including variations in dental eruption or alveolar growth, inordinate neuromuscular growth, and aberrant neuromuscular function because of tongue dysfunction or oral habits [20].

Treatment for this malocclusion is challenging and demands long-term retention. Among the two types of open bite (skeletal and dental open bite), only the open bite of dental origin can be restored by prosthetic rehabilitation [21, 22].

In cases with open bite occlusion, feldspathic veneers may be assumed as a conservative therapy to offer a satisfactory smile. Given the cohesive strength of feldspathic ceramic, Mc Lean has suggested limiting the amount of unsupported ceramic to 2.0 mm to minimize cohesive ceramic fracture. According to Castelnuovo et al., when utilizing a leucite reinforced ceramic like IPS-Empress, the amount of unsupported incisal ceramic can be increased by up to 4.0 mm [19]. The diagnostic wax-up is used to determine how much ceramic should be added to fix an open bite. Some parameters should be taken into consideration, including tooth size, axial inclination, gingival level, tooth-tooth relationships, embrasures, and gingival architecture [20].

If the amount of unsupported incisal ceramic is less than or equal to 4.0 mm, ceramic veneers may be recommended. Instead, zirconia-based crowns may be used when there is more than 4.0 mm of unsupported incisal ceramic because of their superior esthetics and high stress resistance [11].

However, in some cases of severe open bite, complete restoration of the open bite would result in longer incisors than the tooth length recorded by G.V. Black [23]. In order to lessen the dark space between the maxillary and mandibular anterior teeth and enhance esthetics, a partial correction of the open bite will be planned.

7. Crossbite

Anterior crossbite is characterized by an abnormal labiolingual relationship between one or more maxillary and mandibular incisors affecting function and esthetics. In some clinical situations, a fixed prosthesis may be used in place of orthodontic repositioning [24, 25].

Porcelain veneers are contraindicated for the restoration of cross-bited teeth as they can be fractured and debonded due to the excessive stress [26]. A more aggressive approach to tooth preparation and full coverage crowns are required to address this malocclusion.

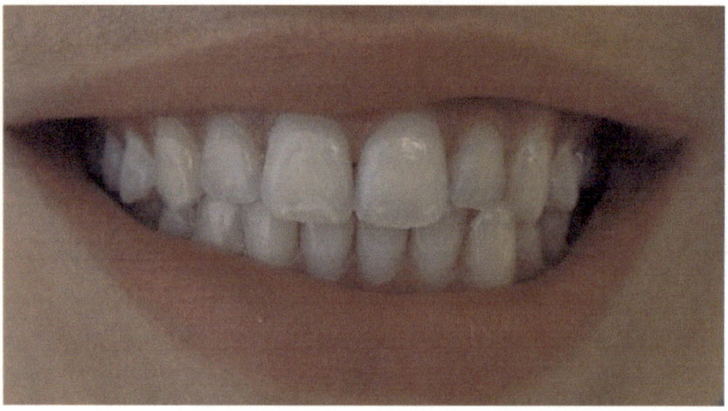

Figure 10.
Anterior crossbite.

Changes in the proprioception of the teeth and lips must be taken into account when treating an anterior crossbite (**Figure 10**). Enough alveolar bone is necessary to support the new tooth position in an anterior crossbite. Since the strains are reversed, the alveolar bone and periodontal ligament will realign to the new stresses [27].

8. Deep bite

Deep bite is one of the most challenging malocclusions to treat successfully. According to Bishara, a deep bite is a malocclusion in which the maxillary incisors excessively overlap the mandibular incisor crowns vertically when the teeth are in centric occlusion [28]. Lack of inter-occlusal space, soft tissue trauma, and tooth wear are among the complications that are caused by the deep overbite. As a result, restorative management may be necessary and could involve extending the occlusal vertical dimension with fixed restorations. To create prostheses with the appropriate functional and occlusal context, careful assessment and treatment planning are, therefore, imperative.

Study models should be articulated on a semi-adjustable articulator in order to plan treatment. Models' articulation makes it easier to evaluate occlusal interactions and can aid in figuring out how much more OVD is required to provide the conceivable treatment. Dentate patients tolerate well OVD changes. The limitations of this approach have been identified by a number of authors, who demonstrated that most therapies may be delivered with increments of between 1 and 3 mm. The diagnostic wax-up with elevated OVD can aid in treatment planning. To safeguard weaker teeth, the occlusal morphology of anterior restorations must be carefully studied, and the proper wax-up guidance should be produced [20].

9. The choices of prosthetic restorations types

9.1 Dental veneers

Dental Veneers present the most conservative prosthetic solution dealing with minor tooth malposition. Once the preparation is performed in the enamel tissue, this therapeutic option should be preferred by the clinician.

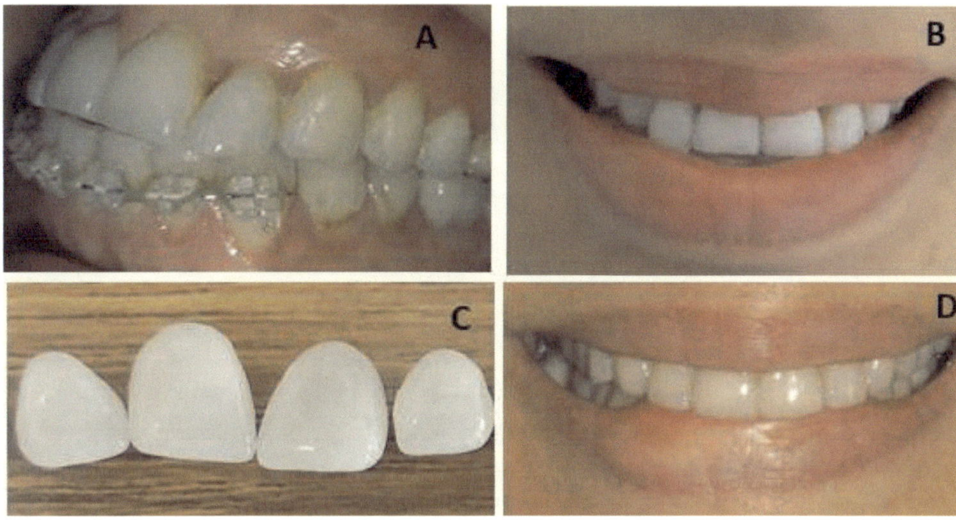

Figure 11.
Clinical situation treated by dental veneers; a: Initial situation showing the anterior gap; B: Initial smile; C: Lithium disilicate ceramic veneers fabricated using chairside CAD/CAM; D: Final outcome with a corrected open bite.

The present clinical situation (**Figure 11**) is about a young patient who has already benefited from orthodontic treatment for 4 years. She is not satisfied with the result. She consulted for the correction of a persistent slight gap.

Once the needed preparation was not necessary, four lithium disilicate ceramic veneers were indicated to establish a correct open bite while optimizing the teeth shape and color.

9.2 Full coverage crowns

In some situation where the Dental Veneers cannot be indicated to correct the tooth malposition, full coverage crowns seem to be the most suitable solution.

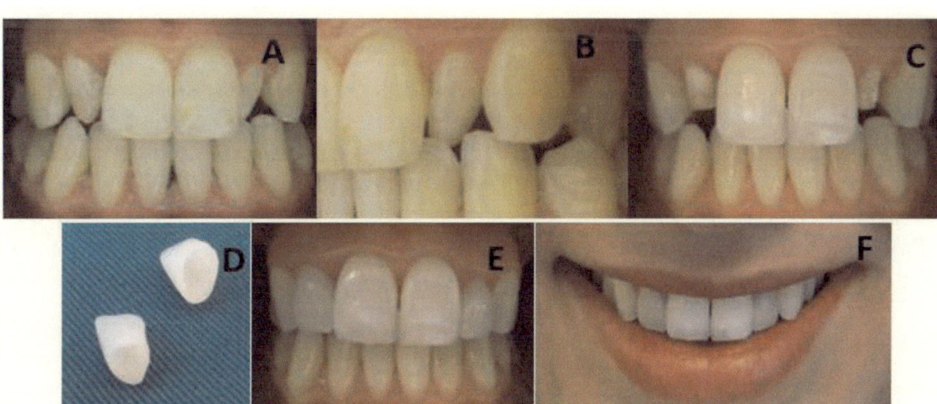

Figure 12.
Clinical situation treated by full coverage crowns; a: Initial situation showing peg-shaped lateral incisors; B: Lateral incisors were in palatal position; C: Prepared teeth; D: Ceramic crowns; E: Final result; F: Final smile.

Clinical situation			Crown	Veneer	Orthodontic treatment
Tooth malposition	Crowding teeth	Score 1	×	×	×
		Score 2	×		×
	Open bite	Minor open bite		×	×
		Severe open bite	×		×
	Crossbite		×		×
	Deep bite		×	×	×

Table 1.
Management of tooth malposition.

The present clinical situation is about a young female patient who asked to regain her smile, judged unsightly, because of peg-shaped maxillary lateral incisors (**Figure 12**). These teeth were, also, in palatal position. After a deep clinical examination, it was decided to perform two IPS e.max CAD crowns.

9.3 What is the suitable prosthetic solution for tooth malposition?

Variable prosthetic solutions are available to manage the tooth malposition.

On the one hand, veneers are the most conservative solution mainly indicated for intact teeth with very slight malposition in order to preserve the enamel tissue necessary for the bonding. Therefore, with the advances in dental ceramics and adhesive systems, porcelain veneers are considered as a much more conservative treatment in terms of preparation, they give satisfactory and lasting esthetic results and they have shown a very important survival rate [14, 29]. Edelhoff and Sorensen measured, with a gravimetric analysis, the amount of tooth structure removed during different preparation designs for many types of prostheses. They showed that tooth preparation for porcelain laminate veneers required approximately one-quarter to one-half the amount of tooth reduction of conventional full coverage crowns [30].

On the other hand, full coverage restorations could be, in some situations, a suitable solution for the management of tooth malposition, as they offer the best solutions in terms of esthetic result, durability, and biocompatibility [29]. But, this type of restoration involves the sacrifice of significant quantities of mineralized dental tissue and cannot be undertaken before the maturation of the periodontal tissues.

Many factors have to be taken into consideration: A deep medical and dental histories, clinical photographs, study casts, periapical and panorama radiographs, the diagnostic wax-up/mock-up, as well as, the use of a planning technique like the digital smile design (DSD).

Table 1 summarizes different solutions managing tooth malposition taking into consideration the open bite, crossbite and deep bite (**Table 1**).

10. Conclusion

The anterior tooth malposition is a frequent chief complaint. The orthodontic treatment is considered as the ideal treatment for those situations. Nevertheless, prosthetic management could be indicated such as dental veneers and full coverage crowns. The most suitable prosthetic solution has to be well raised taking into consideration variable factors to ensure both patient satisfaction and the longevity of this restoration.

Acknowledgements

The authors would like to thank their colleagues from the department of fixed prosthodontics who provided insight and expertise that greatly assisted this chapter book.

Conflict of interest

The authors declare no conflicts of interest.

Author details

Yosra Gassara[1]*, Rim Kallala[1], Emna Boudabous[2], Ines Azouzi[1] and Zohra Nouira[3]

1 Faculty of Dental Medicine of Monastir, Department of Fixed Prosthodontics, Monastir, Tunisia

2 Faculty of Dental Medicine of Monastir, Department of Fixed Prosthodontics, Tunisia

3 Department of Fixed Prosthodontics, Research Laboratory of Occlusodontics and Ceramic Prosthesis LR16ES15, Faculty of Dental Medicine, University of Monastir, Monastir, Tunisia

*Address all correspondence to: chouchengassarayosra@gmail.com

References

[1] Dehghani M, Fazeli F, Sattarzadeh AP. Efficiency and duration of orthodontic/Orthognathic surgery treatment. The Journal of Craniofacial Surgery. 2017;**28**(8):1997-2000

[2] Jacobson N, Frank CA. The myth of instant orthodontics: An ethical quandary. Journal of the American Dental Association (1939). 2008;**139**(4): 424-434

[3] Prakash V, Gupta R. Instant orthodontics – A modality to correct mal-aligned teeth. Journal of Clinical and Diagnostic Research. 2010;**4**:2967-2970

[4] American Dental Association. Principles of Ethics and Code of Professional Conduct, with Official Advisory Opinions, Revised to February 2018. Chicago: ADA; 2018

[5] Urzal V. Relationships between teeth and adjacent structures: How to achieve more esthetic results. International Orthodontics. 2010;**8**(2):91-104

[6] Ward DH. Proportional smile design: Using the recurring Esthetic dental proportion to correlate the widths and lengths of the maxillary anterior teeth with the size of the face. Dental Clinics of North America. 2015;**59**(3):623-638

[7] Ke XP, Wang CW, Sun HQ, Yang Y, Luo XY, Liu TS. A quantitative research on clinical parameters of gingival contour for anterior teeth esthetic analysis and design. Journal of Esthetic and Restorative Dentistry. 2018;**30**(6): 532-537

[8] Pawar B, Mishra P, Banga P, Marawar PP. Gingival zenith and its role in redefining esthetics: A clinical study. Journal of Indian Society and Periodontology. 2011;**15**(2):135-138

[9] Ward DH. Proportional smile design using the recurring esthetic dental (red) proportion. Dental Clinics of North America. 2001;**45**(1): 143-154

[10] Thomas D, Hari K, Mathew J, Bhaskaran S. Esthetic correction with laminate veneers. RRJDS/Aesthetic Restoration-S1. 2017;**6**:21-26

[11] Gurrea J, Bruguera A. Wax-up and mock-up. A guide for anterior periodontal and restorative treatments. Int. Journal of Esthetic Dentistry. 2014; **9**(2):146-162

[12] Jacopo C. Porcelain laminate veneers : Criteria for predictability. Rev Odont Stomat. 2008;**37**:287-315

[13] Cattoni F, Mastrangelo F, Gherlone EF, Gastaldi G. A New Total Digital Smile Planning Technique (3D-DSP) to Fabricate CAD-CAM Mockups for Esthetic Crowns and Veneers. International Journal of Dentistry. 2016; **2016**:1-5

[14] Veneziani M. Ceramic laminate veneers: Clinical procedures with a multidisciplinary approach. International Journal of Esthetic Dentistry. 2017;**12**(4):426-448

[15] VanKirk LK, Pennell EH. Assessment of malocclusion in population groups. American Journal of Orthodontics. 1959; **45**(10):752-758

[16] de Andrade OS, Ferreira LA, Hirata R, Rodrigues FP, D'Alpino PH, Di Hipolito V. Esthetic and functional rehabilitation of crowded mandibular anterior teeth using ceramic veneers: A case report. Quintessence International. 2012;**43**(8):661-670

[17] Vlaskalic V, Boyd R. Orthodontic treatment of a mildly crowded malocclusion using the Invisalign system. Australian Orthodontic Journal. 2001;**17**(1):41-46

[18] Sisler ZS. No-preparation veneers: A minimally invasive approach for a naturally Esthetic smile. The Compendium of Continuing Education in Dentistry. 2018;**39**(10):714-720

[19] Savadi RC, Savadi AR, Kumar PS. Crowns to create Esthetics for mal-aligned central incisors: A case report. Journal of Indian Prosthodontic Society. 2011;**11**(2):121-124

[20] Guven S, Karaman T, Unal M, Melek IC. Rehabilitation of open bite with diastema using zirconia ceramic crowns: Case report. Journal of International Dental and Medical Research. 2013;**6**(2):88-91

[21] Parlani S, Patel S. Esthetic correction in open bite. Indian Journal of Dental Research. 2011;**22**:580-582

[22] Admala SR, Admala NR, Surender LR, Aravelli S. Complete anterior open bite of an adult treated with prosthetic rehabilitation. Journal of Interdisciplinary Dentistry. 2014;**4**: 93-96

[23] Kim S-Y, Lim S-H, Gang S-N, Kim H-J. Crown and root lengths of incisors, canines, and premolars measured by cone-beam computed tomography in patients with malocclusions. Korean. Journal of Orthodontics. 2013;**43**(6):271-278

[24] Esteves H, Correia A. Clinical showcase–correction of an anterior crossbite with a fixed partial denture. Journal of the Canadian Dental Association. 2008; **74**(9):791-794

[25] Bayrak S, Tunc ES. Treatment of anterior dental crossbite using bonded resin-composite slopes: Case reports. Eur. Journal of Dentistry. 2008;**2**(4): 303-306

[26] Jankar AS, Kale Y, Kangane S, Ambekar A, Sinha M, Chaware S. Comparative evaluation of fracture resistance of ceramic veneer with three different incisal design preparations - an In-vitro study. Journal of International Oral Health. 2014;**6**(1):48-54

[27] Madhu S. Preformed stainless steel crown in special conditions in adults: Two case reports. Indian Journal of Dental Research. 2015;**26**:435-438

[28] Daokar S, Agrawal G. Deep bite its etiology, diagnosis and management: A review. Journal of Orthodontics & Endodontics. 2016;**2**:4

[29] Chafaie A. Esthetic management of anterior dental anomalies: A clinical case. International Orthodontics. 2016;**14**(3): 357-365

[30] Edelhoff D, Sorensen JA. Tooth structure removal associated with various preparation designs for anterior teeth. The Journal of Prosthetic Dentistry. 2002;**87**(5):503-509

Chapter 5

Advances in Dentures: Novel Polymeric Materials and Manufacturing Technologies

Lavinia Cosmina Ardelean, Laura-Cristina Rusu, Codruta Victoria Tigmeanu, Meda Lavinia Negrutiu and Daniela Maria Pop

Abstract

Acrylic resins dominated dentures technology for several decades. Due to their many disadvantages, new types of polymers, with better properties, suitable for dental prosthodontics applications were constantly attempted. The choice of polymeric materials and manufacturing technologies has experienced significant development in recent years. Different types of thermoplastic injected resins, light-cured resins, or the versatile high-performance polymers are several choices of novel materials for dentures manufacturing. CAD/CAM systems, both substractive and additive, are being considered the most promising choice for the future manufacturing of polymers in dentistry. The chapter is focused on presenting the choices of novel polymeric materials, their manufacturing technologies, and applications in prosthodontics.

Keywords: prosthodontics, high-performance polymers, polyaryletherketone, polyetheretherketone, polyetherketoneketone, PAEK, PEEK, PEKK, acrylic resin, PMMA, polyoxymethylene, acetal, polyurethane, polyamide, thermoplastic, injection, light-curing, CAD/CAM, 3D printing, 4D printing

1. Introduction

Polymer-based materials play an important role in prosthodontics. They have a wide range of applications, including fixed or removable partial dentures, full dentures, overdentures, provisionals, facial prostheses, splints, and mouthguards. The most commonly used polymers in prosthodontics are polymethyl methacrylate (PMMA), polycarbonate (PC), polyurethane (PU), polyamide (PA), polyoxymethylene (POM), and polyaryletherketone (PAEK) [1]. The PAEK family includes polyetheretherketone (PEEK) and polyetherketoneketone (PEKK), both used in prosthodontics.

Due to the fact synthetic PEEK has been recently investigated as an implant material [2, 3], its area of application has expanded to implantology, as well.

Acrylic resins, which represented an important step forward in dentistry, have been used in prosthodontics since the middle of the twentieth century. The drawbacks of classic acrylic resins, manufactured by means of the thermopolymerization technique, include high polymerization shrinkage, low mechanical resistance, awkward flasking, and difficult processing. The residual monomer may result in increased porosity, allergenic potential, and cytotoxicity. Another disadvantage is due to water sorption, which is a slow process and takes place while wearing the denture for a certain period of time, potentially leading to bacterial colonization. Their main advantage is represented by the affordable cost [4, 5]. New classes of acrylics, with better characteristics are currently available, such as thermoplastic, injected, or CAD/CAM manufactured resins.

Concurrently, not only new polymeric materials, with better properties were developed, but also new manufacturing technologies, such as injection, light-curing, CAD/CAM milling, and 3D printing, have emerged.

Thermoplastic (injected) and CAD/CAM manufactured acrylic prosthodontics are being characterized by better impact resistance, long-term stability, and dense and smooth surface, with low or no porosity. Due to the limited water sorption, their long-term stability is higher, and the absence of residual monomers results in good biocompatibility [6].

2. Novel polymeric materials and manufacturing technologies for prosthodontics applications

2.1 Thermoplastic injected polymers

The most used thermoplastic-injected polymers for prosthodontics manufacturing include PA, POM, PMMA, and PAEK. The material, in granular form, wrapped in special cartridges, is heated and injected by means of special devices, excluding any chemical reaction, thus preventing polymerization shrinkage (**Figure 1**) [7, 8].

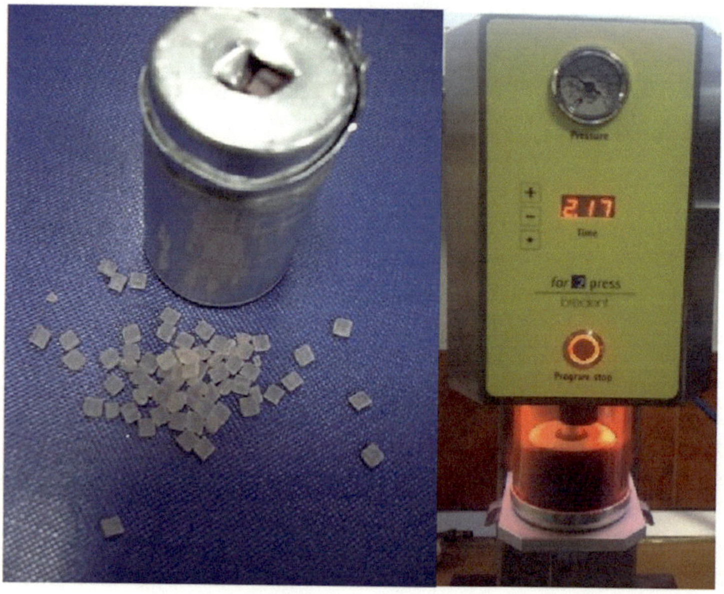

Figure 1.
Thermoplastic polymer for injection, in a granular form; injection unit for thermoplastic resins.

Thermoplastic injected dental polymers are monomer-free, thus nontoxic and biocompatible [9].

They are indicated for manufacturing of removable partial dentures, preformed clasps, removable partial denture frameworks, provisionals, full dentures, orthodontic appliances, anti-snoring devices, mouthguards, and splints [10].

Polyamides are flexible thermoplastics, practically unbreakable, indicated for denture bases in patients with allergies, and retentive dental fields. Based on the flexibility degree, polyamides are classified in superflexible and with medium-low flexibility. The superflexible type is extremely elastic (**Figure 2**), while the medium-low one is a half-soft comfortable material. The clasps may be manufactured from the same material, ready-made clasps may be used, or even metal clasps may be considered (**Figure 2**) [11].

Polyoxymethylene or acetal resins, characterized by low elasticity and high impact strength, are being indicated for replacing the metal framework and clasps in removable partial dentures. Other indications include provisionals, splints, orthodontic appliances, and Kemeny-type single unilateral partial dentures (**Figure 3**).

2.2 Light-cured polymers

Light-cured diacrylic composite resins were initially elaborated as direct esthetic restorative materials, and the indirect type, successfully used in dental laboratories, has been subsequently developed. Their indications include veneering of metal-polymeric crowns and bridges, single-tooth or temporary crowns, inlays, onlays, and repairing damaged porcelain veneers. One of their advantages is the prolonged handling time, as well as good adherence to the metal framework, and low polymerization shrinkage. In certain cases, more than one curing method is used, for example, combination of heat, pressure, and light-curing [12].

The light-curing eclipse resin system (Dentsply-DeguDent) enables the manufacturing of full dentures, removable partial dentures, and splints and allows speedy manufacturing by eliminating time-consuming stages such as pattern modeling, investing, and heat-curing. Composed of three wax-like urethane-based resins: baseplate resin, setup resin, and contour resin, it has no allergic potential.

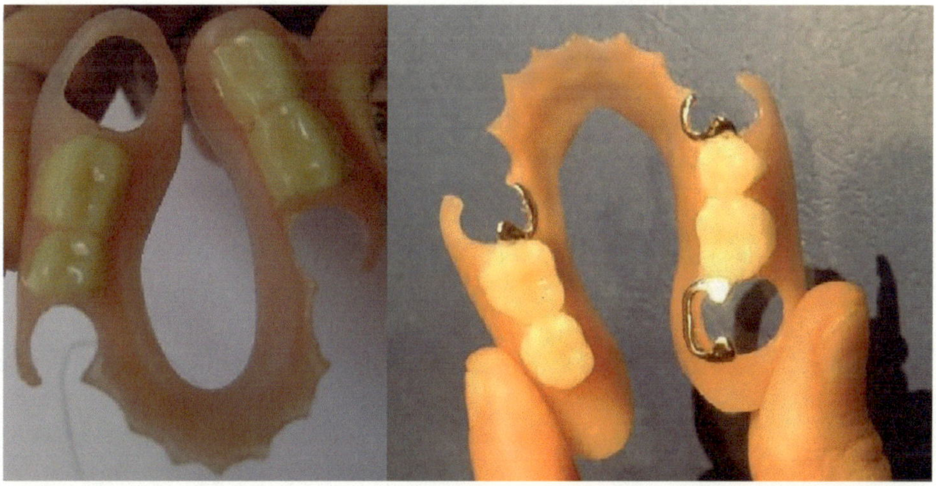

Figure 2.
Superflexible polyamide removable partial denture; superflexible polyamide removable partial denture combined with metal clasps.

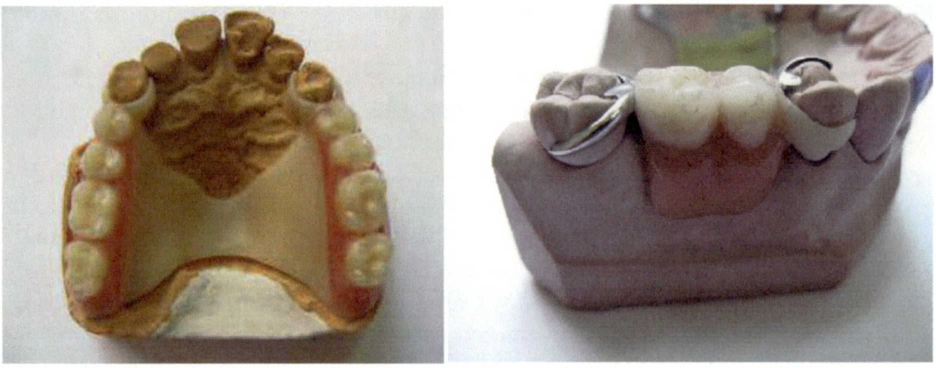

Figure 3.
Removable partial dentures with POM framework and clasps, and PMMA saddles; combination between a thermoplastic PMMA resin saddle, metal, and POM clasps.

The first step is mounting the teeth directly on the denture's light-cured base. The denture itself is used for try-in, and the esthetic and phonetic checking is being carried out. Afterwards, the setup and contour resins are used to finalize the denture, which is light-cured (**Figures 4–6**) [13, 14].

2.3 CAD/CAM manufactured polymers

CAD/CAM systems, either substractive or additive, have been used in dentistry since 1980s, at first for fixed prosthodontic restorations, later on, expanding to removable prosthodontic restorations, as well as various dental appliances [15].

CAD/CAM systems have three major components. The data acquisition may be carried out by intraoral or extraoral scanning. Extraoral scanning involves data acquisition by means of an impression or a model, which is being converted into virtual models. The second component is the software. Its role is to design the virtual restorations and establish the milling parameters. The third component depends on the type of the system, substractive or additive. A milling machine is used for substractive from a material block (**Figure 7**). 3D printing device is used for additive manufacturing [16].

The advantages of CAD/CAM systems are reduced number of appointments and the ease to access the previously saved digital data if needed [17].

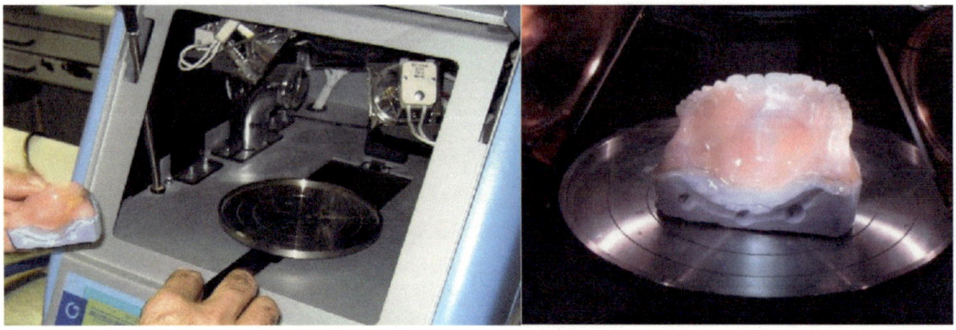

Figure 4.
Light curing of the denture base and of the finalized denture.

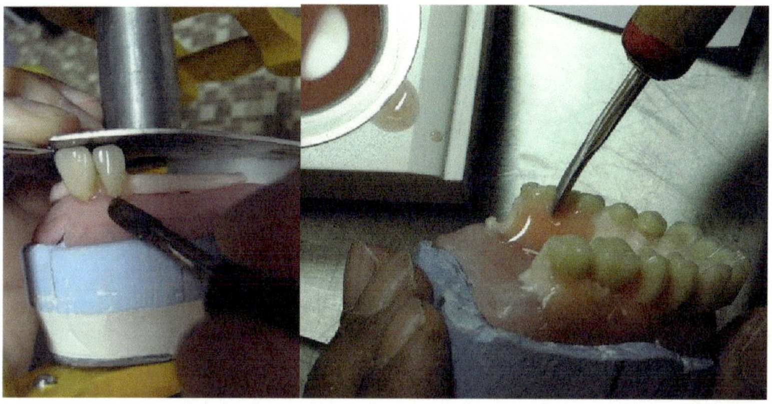

Figure 5.
Teeth mounting on the denture's light-cured base, by using the setup resin.

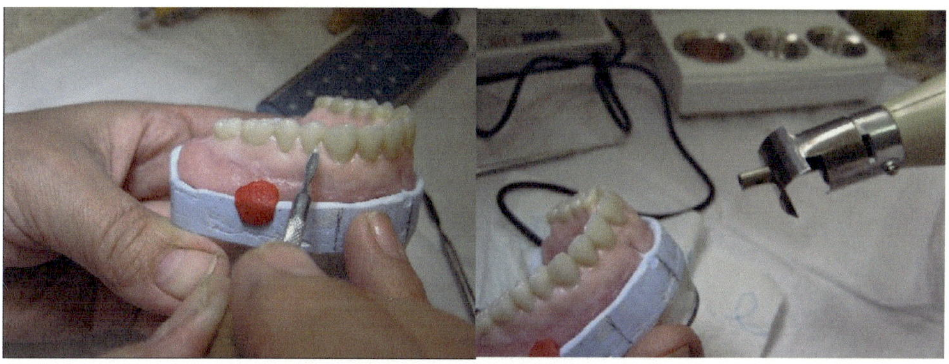

Figure 6.
Applying the contour resin, and processing it by using the warm air gun to create a smooth surface.

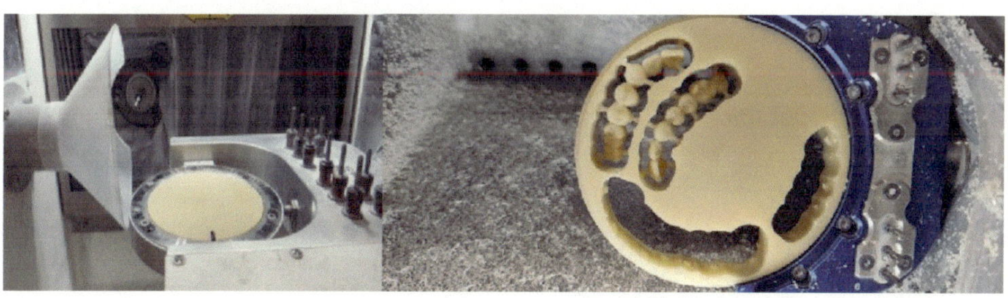

Figure 7.
PMMA block; milling artificial teeth from a PMMA block.

The high initial cost of the milling machine or 3D printing device may be overcome by referring the data to a milling or 3D printing center, which will handle the manufacturing step.

The most used polymeric materials for CAD/CAM milling are PMMA, composite resins, PU, PC, and PEEK. It is major indications for polymeric materials include provisionals, crowns, copings, mouthguards, short bridges, veneers, inlays, onlays, denture bases, artificial teeth, removable partial dentures framework and clasps, patterns, and models. The bicolored discs allow manufacturing of monolithic total dentures in one uninterrupted milling process.

Probably, the most important advantage of the subtractive method is using homogenous materials. However, its major drawback is due to material loss which leads to higher costs.

The additive manufacturing addresses these drawbacks in the CAM step, and the prosthodontic devices being fabricated by materials layering [18]. The materials present themselves in different forms, depending on the type of 3D printing method used.

The most frequently used 3D printing methods for dental polymers are based on vat photo-polymerization, material jetting, and material extrusion, showing noticeable differences in resolution, accuracy, and repeatability [19].

Currently, vat photo-polymerization technologies are the most used in dentistry, including the stereolithography (SLA) and digital light processing (DLP) methods. The material, in a liquid form, is being selectively light-cured by means of a directed UV-laser beam (SLA) or a UV-light mask (DLP) (**Figure 8**). Unluckily, both SLA and DLP printed objects need post-processing. The post-processing steps include cleaning with isopropanol, to remove the residual monomer, and post-polymerization (**Figure 9**) [20–22].

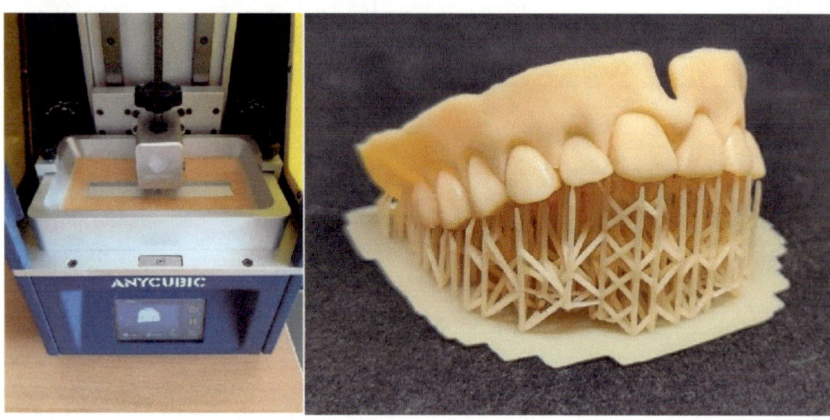

Figure 8.
SLA 3D printer; 3D printed dental model.

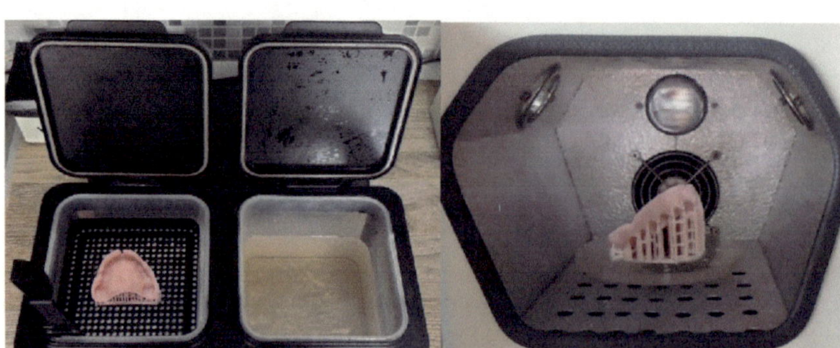

Figure 9.
Post-processing of a SLA 3D printed denture base: Cleaning with isopropanol, and post-polymerization.

Both SLA and DLP allow manufacturing a wide selection of polymeric materials: PMMA, reinforced PMMA, Bis-GMA, and UDMA-based resins, PU [23].

Material jetting (MJT) is a droplet-based and photo-polymerization technique. The material, in a liquid form, is applied, as tiny drops, from the print head directly to the build platform, and needs no post-processing. The layer-by-layer deposition is extremely fast and highly accurate. A special feature of MJT is the possibility of multi-material, multicolor 3D printing [23].

Fusion deposition modeling (FDM) is an extrusion-based printing technique. Thermoplastic materials, in a filament form, are being deposited layer-by-layer [24].

A wide range of thermoplastic polymeric materials, including polyesters, PA, PU, PC, acrylonitrile butadiene styrene, and PEEK are being used.

MJT and FDM also allow a multi-material, multicolor 3D printing mode.

The applications of 3D printing include models, custom trays, dental bites, provisionals, crowns, full dentures, removable partial dentures frameworks and clasps, artificial teeth, try-ins, surgical/implant guides, templates, implants, orthodontic appliances, and mouthguards. Flexible polymers may be used to manufacture 3Dprinted dentures bases and mouthguards [18].

2.4 Shape memory 4D printed polymers

4D printing, incorporating time as the fourth dimension, enables printing constructs, which are capable to transform over time, under different stimuli, allowing the creation of complicated structures with on-demand dynamically controllable shapes and functions (**Figure 10**) [25]. Shape memory polymers are capable of remembering permanent shapes, present the capability to be deformed temporally, and return to their original shape under an external stimulus [26].

4D printing has proven its efficiency in dentistry due to the dynamic oral environment, which undergoes continuous changes of temperature and humidity [27].

4D printed denture bases adapt to the occlusion forces, including eating and drinking patterns, and are being characterized by similar elasticity and thermal properties as the oral tissues. In the case of residual ridge resorption, using smart materials to compensate for bone loss has been attempted. Other applications of 4D printing in prosthodontics include crown copings, removable partial dentures frameworks, orthodontic appliances, surgical guides, and implants [28].

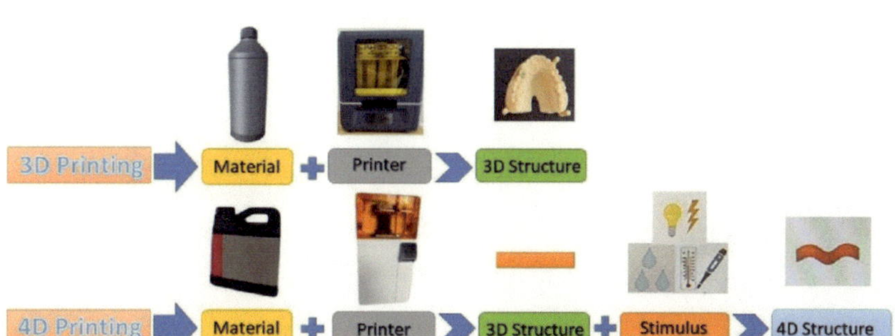

Figure 10.
Comparative schematics of 3D and 4D printing technologies.

2.5 High-performance polymers

High-performance polymers are characterized by the capability to preserve their mechanical, thermal, and chemical properties when submitted to various extreme environmental conditions [29].

The most used high-performance polymers for dental application are PEEK and PEKK-based, both belonging to the PAEK family. PEEK and PEKK are ketone-based, thermoplastic polymers, with excellent mechanical and chemical resistance, and low water sorption, being highly biocompatible, and displaying an elasticity comparable to bone [30]. Compared to acrylic resins, PAEK has no residual monomer content and has no allergenic potential. Due to its corrosion resistance, PAEK is considered as an alternative to metallic restorations. It has the advantage to be lightweight (**Figure 11**), but, because of its opacity and whitish-gray color, needs to be veneered, when used for fixed restorations. Because of its bone-like elasticity module, it is considered a good option for Ti implants.

Its indications include copings, bridges infrastructure, removable partial dentures framework and clasps, implants, and implant abutments (**Figures 12** and **13**). It may be optimized by adding ceramic or hydroxyapatite nanoparticles and carbon fibers [31, 32].

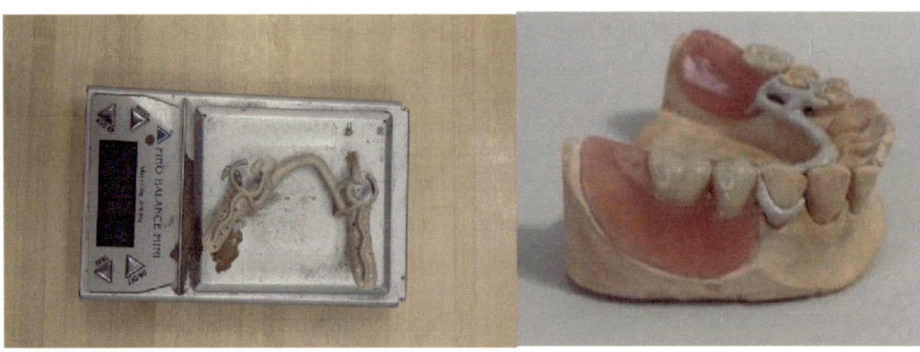

Figure 11.
A milled removable partial denture framework, made of PEEK (including clasps), weight only 1.36 grams. The removable partial denture, including the acrylic saddles, weight only 3.36 grams.

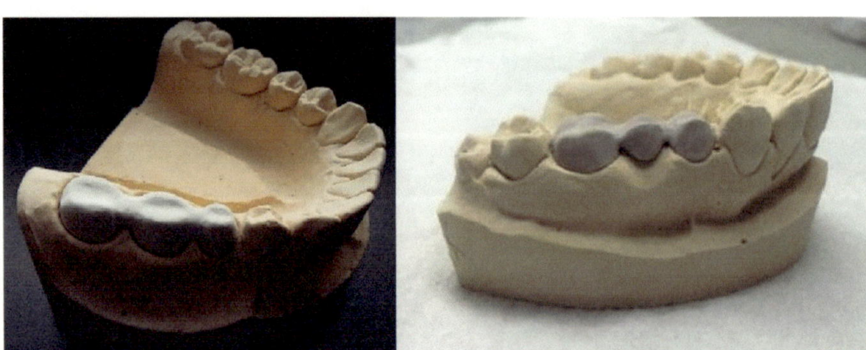

Figure 12.
PEEK and PEKK bridge infrastructures, respectively.

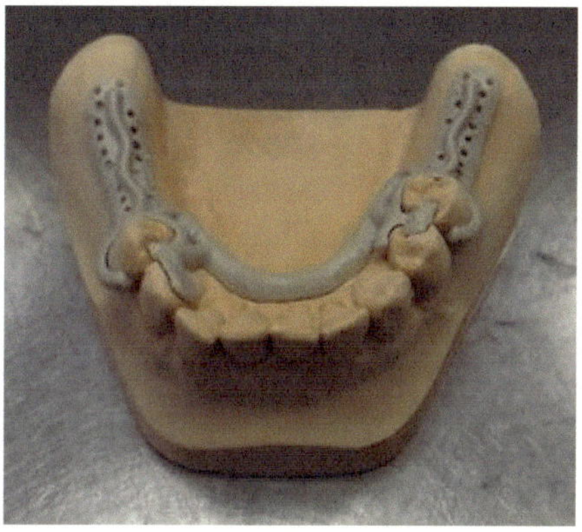

Figure 13.
PEEK removable partial denture framework and clasps.

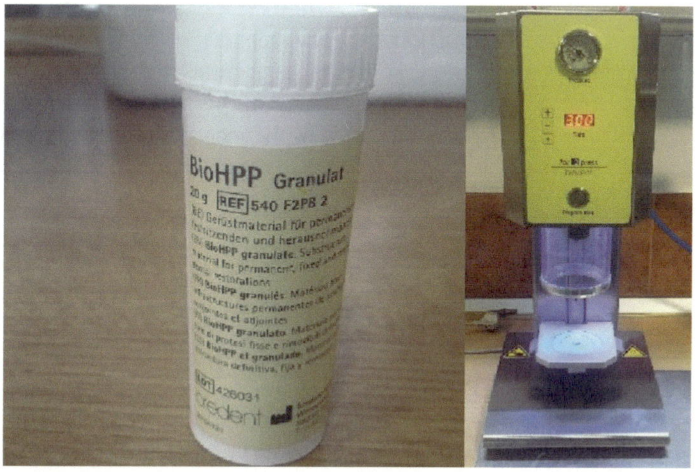

Figure 14.
PEEK in granular form and the injection unit.

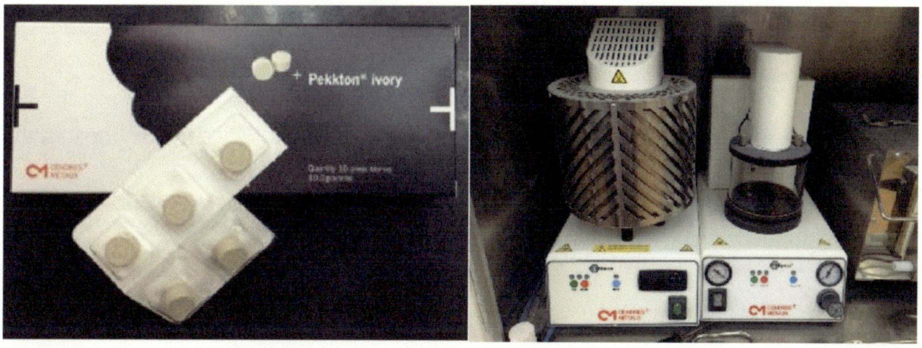

Figure 15.
PEKK ingots, the preheating, and the injection units.

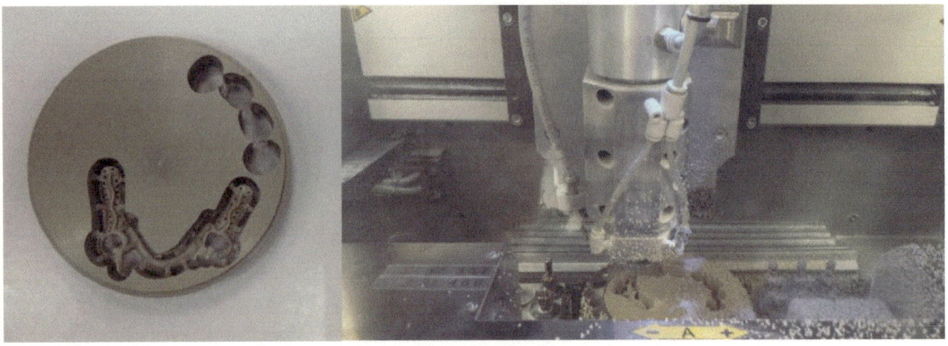

Figure 16.
PEEK block for CAD/CAM milling; milling of a PEEK block.

In the case of PEEK implants, because the material is bioinert, it lacks osseointegration, so coating is needed [2, 33]. PEEK is also considered a choice for scaffold manufacture, despite its non-degradability, when blended with biodegradable polymers, such as poly(glycolic acid) and polyvinyl alcohol [34, 35].

PEEK in granular form and PEKK in ingots form may be manufactured by injection (**Figures 14** and **15**). PEEK and PAEK blocks are being used for milling by CAD/CAM substractive systems, (**Figure 16**), and, more recently, PEEK in a filament form has been used for 3D printing, namely by FDM, or SLS, which uses the material in a powder form [36, 37].

3. Conclusion

Multiple options of novel polymeric materials for prosthodontic applications are currently available. Various technologies have been attempted to replace the classic thermopolymerization method used for PMMA dentures. Each material and technology has its advantages and drawbacks, and the best choice should be made considering the status of the patient, the available technological infrastructure, and the involved costs. The future in prosthetics comes with the emerging new smart polymeric materials, which are able to self-adapt in the continuously changing conditions of the oral environment.

Acknowledgements

The authors would like to thank Professor Cristina-Maria Bortun for her valuable contribution and support.

Conflict of interest

The authors declare no conflict of interest.

Author details

Lavinia Cosmina Ardelean[1*], Laura-Cristina Rusu[2], Codruta Victoria Tigmeanu[1], Meda Lavinia Negrutiu[3] and Daniela Maria Pop[3]

1 Department of Technology of Materials and Devices in Dental Medicine, Multidisciplinary Center for Research, Evaluation, Diagnosis and Therapies in Oral Medicine, "Victor Babes" University of Medicine and Pharmacy Timisoara, Timisoara, Romania

2 Department of Oral Pathology, Multidisciplinary Center for Research, Evaluation, Diagnosis and Therapies in Oral Medicine, "Victor Babes" University of Medicine and Pharmacy Timisoara, Timisoara, Romania

3 Department of Prostheses Technology and Dental Materials, Research Center in Dental Medicine Using Conventional and Alternative Technologies, "Victor Babes" University of Medicine and Pharmacy Timisoara, Timisoara, Romania

*Address all correspondence to: lavinia_ardelean@umft.ro

References

[1] Soygun K, Bolayir G, Boztug A. Mechanical and thermal properties of polyamide versus reinforced PMMA denturebase materials. The Journal of Advanced Prosthodontics. 2013;**5**: 153-160. DOI: 10.4047/jap.2013.5.2.153

[2] Najeeb S, Zafar MS, Khurshid Z, Siddiqui F. Applications of polyetheretherketone (PEEK) in oral implantology and prosthodontics. Journal of Prosthodontic Research. 2016;**60**:12-19. DOI: 10.1016/j.jpor.2015.10.001

[3] Al-Rabab'ah M, Hamadneh W, Alsalem I, Khraisat A, Karaky AA. Use of high performance polymers as dental implant abutments and frameworks: A case series report. Journal of Prosthodontics. 2019;**28**:365-372. DOI: 10.1111/jopr.12639

[4] Gautam R, Singh RD, Sharma VP, Siddartha R, Chand P, Kumar R. Biocompatibility of polymethylmethacrylate resins used in dentistry. Journal of Biomedical Materials Research Part B Applied Biomaterials. 2012;**100B**:1444-1450. DOI: 10.1002/jbm.b.32673

[5] Takahashi Y, Yoshida K, Shimizu H. Fracture resistance of maxillary complete dentures subjected to long term water immersion. Gerodontology. 2012;**29**:e1086-e1091. DOI: 10.1111/j.1741-2358.2012.00616.x

[6] Ardelean L, Bortun CM, Podariu AC, Rusu LC. Acrylates and their alternatives in dental applications. In: Reddy BSR, editor. Acrylic Polymers in Healthcare. London: IntechOpen; 2017. pp. 3-24. DOI: 10.5772/66610

[7] Fueki K, Ohkubo C, Yatabe M, Arakawa I, Arita M, et al. Clinical application of removable partial dentures using thermoplastic resin. Part I: Definition and indication of non-metal clasp dentures. Journal of Prosthodontic Research. 2014;**58**:3-10. DOI: 10.1016/j.jpor.2013.12.002

[8] Fueki K, Ohkubo C, Yatabe M, Arakawa I, Arita M, Ino S, et al. Clinical application of removable partial dentures using thermoplastic resin. Part II: Material properties and clinical features of non-metal clasp dentures. Journal of Prosthodontic Research. 2014;**58**:71-84. DOI: 10.1016/j.jpor.2014.03.002

[9] Nakhaei M, Dashti H, Barazandeh R, et al. Shear bond strength of acrylic denture teeth to PMMA and polyamide denture base material. Journal of Dental Materials and Techniques. 2018;**7**:19-23. DOI: 10.22038/JDMT.2017.10003

[10] Ardelean L, Bortun CM, Podariu AC, Rusu LC. Thermoplastic resins used in dentistry. In: Das CK, editor. Thermoplastic Elastomers. Synthesis and Applications. Rijeka: InTech; 2015. pp. 145-167. DOI: 10.5772/59647

[11] Yunus N, Rashid AA, Azmi LL, Abu-Hassan MI. Some flexural properties of a nylon denture base polymer. Journal of Oral Rehabilitation. 2005;**32**:65-71. DOI: 10.1111/j.1365-2842.2004.01370.x

[12] Bortun CM, Ardelean L, Rusu LC, Marcauteanu C. Importance of modern light-curing resins in the design of removable partial dentures. Revista de Chimie. 2012;**63**:428-431

[13] Kurtzman GM, Melton AB. Full arch removable prosthetics with eclipse. Spectrum Denturism. 2008;**2**:1-8

[14] Bortun C, Cernescu A, Ghiban N, Faur N, Ghiban B, Gombos O, et al.

Durability evaluation of complete dentures realized with "eclipse prosthetic resin system". Revista Materiale Plastice. 2010;**47**:457-460

[15] Sen N, Us YO. Mechanical and optical properties of monolithic CAD-CAM restorative materials. Journal of Prosthetic Dentistry. 2018;**119**:593-599. DOI: 10.1016/j.prosdent.2017.06.-12

[16] Abdullah AO, Muhammed FK, Zheng B, Liu Y. An overview of computer aided design/computer aided manufacturing (CAD/CAM) in restorative dentistry. Journal of Dental Materials and Techniques. 2018;7:1-10. DOI: 10.22038/JDMT.2017.26351.1213

[17] Kattadiyil MT, Al Helal A, Goodacre BJ. Clinical complications and quality assessments with computer-engineered complete dentures: A systematic review. Journal of Prosthetic Dentistry. 2017;**117**:721-728. DOI: 10.1016/j.prosdent.2016.12.006

[18] Tigmeanu CV, Ardelean LC, Rusu LC, Negrutiu ML. Additive manufactured polymers in dentistry, current state-of-the-art and future perspectives-A review. Polymers. 2022;**14**:3658. DOI: 10.3390/polym14173658

[19] Jockusch J, Özcan M. Additive manufacturing of dental polymers: An overview on processes, materials and applications. Dental Materials Journal. 2020;**39**:345-354. DOI: 10.4012/dmj.2019-123

[20] Pillai S, Upadhyay A, Khayambashi P, Farooq I, Sabri H, Tarar M, et al. Dental 3D-printing: Transferring art from the laboratories to the clinics. Polymers. 2021;**13**:157. DOI: 10.3390/polym13010157

[21] Della Bona A, Cantelli V, Britto VT, Collares KF, Stansbury JW. 3D printing restorative materials using a stereolithographic technique: A systematic review. Dental Materials. 2021;**37**:336-350. DOI: 10.1016/j.dental.2020.11.030

[22] Schweiger J, Edelhoff D, Güth J-F. 3D printing in digital prosthetic dentistry: An overview of recent developments in additive manufacturing. Journal of Clinical Medicine. 2021;**10**:2010. DOI: 10.3390/jcm10092010

[23] Theus AS, Ning L, Hwang B, Gil C, Chen S, Wombwell A, et al. Bioprintability: Physiomechanical and biological requirements of materials for 3D bioprinting processes. Polymers. 2020;**1**:2262. DOI: 10.3390/polym12102262

[24] Rebong RE, Stewart KT, Utreja A, Ghoneima AA. Accuracy of three-dimensional dental resin models created by fused deposition modeling, stereolithography, and Polyjet prototype technologies: A comparative study. The Angle Orthodontist. 2018;**88**:363-369. DOI: 10.2319/071117-460.1

[25] Zhang Z, Demir KG, Gu GX. Developments in 4D-printing: A review on current smart materials, technologies, and applications. International Journal of Social Network Mining. 2019;**10**:205-224. DOI: 10.1080/19475411.2019.1591541

[26] Choong YY, Maleksaeedi S, Eng H, Wei J, Su PC. 4D printing of high performance shape memory polymer using stereolithography. Materials & Design. 2017;**126**:219-225. DOI: 10.1016/j.matdes.2017.04.049

[27] Manikandan N, Rajesh PK, Harish V. An analysis of the methods and materials for 4-dimensional printing. Materials Today: Proceedings. 2021;**38**:2167-2173. DOI: 10.1016/j.matpr.2020.05.551

[28] Badami V, Ahuja B. Biosmart materials: Breaking new ground in dentistry. Science World Journal. 2014;**2014**:986912. DOI: 10.1155/2014/986912

[29] Pidhatika B, Widyaya VT, Nalam PC, Swasono YA, Ardhani R. Surface modifications of high-performance polymer Polyetheretherketone (PEEK) to improve its biological performance in dentistry. Polymers. 2022;*14*:5526. DOI: 10.3390/polym14245526

[30] Bathala L, Majeti V, Rachuri N, Singh N, Gedela S. The role of polyether ether ketone (PEEK) in dentistry—A review. Journal of Medicine and Life. 2019;**12**:5-9. DOI: 10.25122/jml-2019-0003

[31] Ichikawa T, Kurahashi K, Liu L, Matsuda T, Ishida Y. Use of a Polyetheretherketone clasp retainer for removable partial dentures: A case report. Dentistry Journal. 2019;**7**:4. DOI: 10.3390/dj7010004

[32] Zoidis P, Papathanasiou I, Polyzois G. The use of a modified poly-ether-ether-ketone (PEEK) as an alternative framework material for removable dental prostheses. A clinical report. Journal of Prosthodontics. 2016;**140**:580-584. DOI: 10.1111/jopr.12325

[33] Rahmitasari F, Ishida Y, Kurahashi K, Matsuda T, Watanabe M, Ichikawa T. PEEK with reinforced materials and modifications for dental implant applications. Dentistry Journal. 2017;**15**:35. DOI: 10.3390/dj5040035

[34] Liao C, Li Y, Tjong SC. Polyetheretherketone and its composites for bone replacement and regeneration. Polymers. 2020;*12*:2858. DOI: 10.3390/polym12122858

[35] Feng P, Jia J, Peng S, Yang W, Bin S, Shuai C. Graphene oxide-driven interfacial coupling in laser 3D printed PEEK/PVA scaffolds for bone regeneration. Virtual and Physical Prototyping. 2020;**15**:211-226. DOI: 10.1080/17452759.2020.1719457

[36] Vaezi M, Yang S. Extrusion-based additive manufacturing of PEEK for biomedical applications. Virtual and Physical Prototyping. 2015;**310**:123-135. DOI: 10.1080/17452759.2015.1097053

[37] Lee CU, Vandenbrande J, Goetz A, Ganter MA, Storti DW, Boydston AJ. Room temperature extrusion 3D printing of poly-ether ether ketone using a stimuli-responsive binder. Additive Manufacturing. 2019;**28**:430-438. DOI: 10.1016/j.addma.2019.05.008

Chapter 6

Reinforced Filler in Denture Base Materials

Saied H. Mohamed

Abstract

Dental prosthesis nowadays fabricated from Poly (methyl methacrylate) (PMMA) due to its easy handling, exceptional appearance. However, this material as an ideal denture base is still restricted by a few limitations such as poor strength and radiopacity. Attempts to improve the mechanical and radiopacity properties of denture base materials through the inclusion of verity of fiber and fillers. A nano-filler modified with the silane coupling agent could improve the dispersiblity of the fillers in polymer matrix. The clinical problem of using silanes in adhesion promotion is bond degradation over time in the oral environment. This chapter presents the fillers as reinforcement agent for improving denture base properties. It reviews different types of fibers and fillers added to PMMA denture base resin and evaluates their effect on the physical and mechanical properties. Comprehensive research in review of literature were carried out included longstanding and update studies in electronic data base including PubMed, Google search, Science Direct and Research Gate. All studies were presented and their finding were discussed. The future of manufacturing applications in 3D printing and CAD/CAM technology of denture base resins with improvement in their properties for 3D printing technology and digital denture base fabrications was also presented.

Keywords: PMMA, denture base, filler, physical and mechanical properties, dental prosthesis

1. Introduction

As dental resins enter into the new era of development, the choice of suitable materials becomes more diverse as they have broadened the range of dental products in all areas of dentistry. Prosthetic dentistry has also broadened its range of many promising materials for denture fabrication. Many different types of materials were used for fabrication of denture base. Prior to 1940, vulcanite was the most widely used denture base polymer. This is a highly cross-linked nature rubber, which is difficult to pigment and tends to become unhygienic due to uptake of saliva. Various other materials have been used in denture construction, including cellulose products, phenol-formaldehyde, vinyl resin, polyamine polymers. However, they have suffered from a variety of problems [1, 2].

In the 1930s, Walter Wright and the Vernon brothers at the Rohm and Haas Company in Philadelphia developed poly (methyl methacrylate) (PMMA), a hard plastic. Although many other materials were utilized for dental prosthetics none could come close to that of PMMA, and nowadays more than 90% of dentures are fabricated from this acrylic polymer [3]. The popularity of PMMA is associated with its favorable working characteristics, processing ease, accurate fit, stability in oral environment, superior esthetics, and use with minimum and inexpensive equipment [4].

This chapter presents a comprehensive review of various fibers and fillers utilized in PMMA denture base resin and their influence on the physical and mechanical properties. The review involves relevant data and sources from scientific papers, reviews, and abstracts published in dental literature. The search for published materials was conducted using both general and specialist databases, such as Google Scholar, Research Gate, and PubMed, with the aid of specific keywords including denture base, PMMA, reinforcement, nanoparticles, fibers, and fillers.

2. The criteria for an ideal denture base material

The requirements of a denture base material can be conveniently categorized into physical, chemical, mechanical, biological, and miscellaneous properties.

2.1 Physical properties

Ideal denture base material should be capable of matching the appearance of the natural oral soft tissue. The importance of this requirement varies considerably, depending on whether the base will be visible when the patient opens his mouth. A polymer, which is used to construct a denture base, ought to have a value of glass transition temperature (Tg), which is high enough to prevent softening and distortion during service. Although the normal temperature in the mouth varies from 32 to 37°C, account must be taken of the fact that patients sometimes take hot drinks higher than this temperature, and also clean their dentures in very hot water despite being advised not to do so.

The base is supposed to have good dimensional stability in order for the shapes of the denture not to change over a period of time. In addition to distortion, which may occur due to thermal softening, other mechanisms such as relief of internal stresses, and water absorption may contribute to dimensional instability. The material should ideally have a low value of specific gravity and dentures should be as light as possible.

The denture base should have radiopaque characteristics leading to its event of detection using normal diagnostic radiographic techniques. Early radiological detection of the denture or fragment of denture is immense help in deciding the best course of treatment.

2.2 Mechanical properties

The denture base should be rigid and has high modulus of elasticity. A high value of elastic limit is required to ensure that stresses encountered during bite and mastication do not cause permanent deformation. It ought to have sufficient flexural strength to resist bending and fracture. The base material should have an adequate fatigue life and high impact strength. Denture base materials need to possess sufficient abrasion and indentation resistance to prevent excessive wear of material by abrasive denture cleaners or foodstuffs.

2.3 Chemical properties

A denture base material should be chemically inert. It should be naturally insoluble in oral fluids and should not absorb water or saliva since this may alter the mechanical properties of the material and cause unhygienic denture.

2.4 Biological properties

In the unmixed or uncured states, the denture base material should not be harmful to the technician involved in its handling. Furthermore, it has to be non-toxic and non-irritant to the patient. The base should neither promote nor sustain the growth of bacteria and fungus.

2.5 Miscellaneous properties

An ideal denture base material ought to be relatively inexpensive and has a long shelf life so that the material can be purchased in bulk and stored without deteriorating. The material should be easy to manipulate and fabricate without having to resort to expensive processing equipment. It should be easy to repair on the occasion of fractures.

2.5.1 Radiopacity of denture base material

Many attempts were tried to achieve the radiopacity into PMMA as denture base material. These efforts include the addition of finely divided metal such as powdered dental amalgam or gold powder, simple halogen-containing molecules such as tetrabromoethane or organo metallic such as triphenly bismuth. Additionally, the incorporation of insoluble inorganic heavy metal salts such as $BaSO_4$, BaF_2, $BiCl_3$, BiBr3, or finely divided glasses containing barium or bismuth [5].

All these techniques exhibit specific disadvantages, which had precluded their use. Out of all the heavy metal inorganic salts and glasses that have been investigated, only $BaSO_4$ has achieved conventional exploitation as an x-ray opacifying agent for both denture base and also as the opacifying medium in methacrylate.

As far as denture base is concerned the resin produced is opaque white and even when tinted, the translucent of nature gum tissue cannot be mimicked so it was never poplar [6]. Moreover, the x-ray opacity was poor and not only simply a question of adding more $BaSO_4$ as not only did the esthetic qualities suffer further but the mechanical properties began to deteriorate as well [5, 6]. There is another radiopacifier described based on iodine-methacrylate, where the contrast agent was introduced via the liquid component and via iodine-containing copolymer [7]. Since the conversion of monomers during curing is incomplete, free monomer will always be present and as a result, there is always a risk for in situ release of iodine-containing methacrylates. Because nothing is known about the toxic effects of such a monomer, this poses an unknown and presumably unacceptable risk for the patient. Therefore, a covalently bound x-ray opacifier would eliminate many of the inherent difficulties that others have found toward the successful development of an x-ray opaque PMMA denture base material.

Lewis et al. [8] studied radiopacifying particle reinforced PMMA. Their approach for enhancing the properties of the polymer and reducing the production of wear particles and debris was directed toward the mechanical reinforcement through the radiopacifier particles. They investigated the improvement of the interface adhesion by establishing covalent chemical bonding between the inorganic fillers (oxide particles) and the PMMA matrix. This was achieved through the preliminary treatment of the fillers surface with a silane bonding agent as 3-(trimethoxysilyl) propyl methacrylate (γ-MPS), capable of later copolymerizing with the (co) monomers.

Abboud et al. [9] studied the mechanical characterization of acrylic resin prepared from γ-MPS treated alumina particles, which could act simultaneously as radiopacifying and reinforcing agents. They found that for some formulations, the compressive strength and modulus reached 150 and 3400 MPa respectively. Those formulations require high concentration of silanated alumina particles (over 35%wt) and such composites are unprocessable due to the lack of liquid monomer for simultaneously wetting the filler surface and dissolving the PMMA beads.

Mohamed [10] studied the ability of HA and alumina in acting as both radiopacifying and reinforcement agents in PMMA denture base material. The effects of the particles microstructures, surface treatment of fillers with γ- MPS were also evaluated. The author concluded that the incorporation of γ- MPS treated ceramic fillers into PMMA matrix in general, has increased the flexural modulus, tensile strength, tensile modulus, and fracture toughness of PMMA denture base material.

2.5.2 Fracture toughness

Fracture toughness is an intrinsic characteristic of a material concerning resistance to crack propagation. It is a measure of the energy required to initiate and propagate a crack in a material, which may lead to catastrophic failure. Fractures are usually classified as brittle fracture and ductile fracture. In brittle fracture, the materials behave elastically up to the point of failure. There is hardly observable deformation of the materials prior or during breakage [11].

The fracture surfaces are relatively smooth and largely perpendicular to the direction of the applied stress. The two surfaces can be fit together quite accurately. Ductile fracture implied that large permanent deformation has occurred before failure, requiring a significant greater amount of energy absorption by the part before failure. Since the result of permanent deformation, the fracture surfaces do not match, and the cross-sectional area at the location of the fracture is reduced from the original value.

The common measurement of fracture toughness is called the critical stress intensity factor (KIC). The KIC is the critical value of material that fracture occurs when an applied stress intensity factor on the material is greater than the critical value. The stress intensity factor K, is a measure of applied stress associated with crack size. When the KIC value is exceeded at the crack tip, the material will then fracture spontaneously leading to complete failure. Below the KIC value the crack can still grow slowly. Because the KIC is measured as stress intensity and not just as a stress, its units are MN/m1.5 [12].

The fracture toughness test is very efficient and other parameters can also be derived from it including modulus of elasticity and the plasticity of the material. The fracture toughness is closely related to fatigue strength [12].

Factors that contribute to stress concentration enable the initiation and propagation of cracks, thereby influencing the rate of failure. As described by Yee [13] the observed energy loss during the impact test depends on four factors; (a) the energy to bend the specimen up to the point of crack initiation, (b) the energy to propagate the crack through the specimen, (c) the kinetic energy of the fractured specimen, and (d) the vibrational or otherwise dissipated energy. As previously reported in the literature, the fracture toughness test appears to be more reliable and advantageous than impact testing when determining the influence of variation in the material composition [14].

Zappini et al. [15] determined the fracture toughness of denture base resins and compared the results with impact strength measurements. Seven heat-polymerized denture base resins were chosen for the study. They concluded that the specimen geometry and testing configuration influenced the impact strength measurements and the fracture toughness method seemed to be more suitable than impact strength measurements to demonstrate the effects of resin modifications. Moreover, the differences between conventional and so-called "high impact" denture base resins were more clearly demonstrated with fracture toughness measurements.

3. Filler reinforced denture base

Reinforcement in particulate denture base may comprise of either flexible particulate rubber, such as in high impact polystyrene (HIPS), or rigid mineral fillers, including hydroxyapatite, alumina calcium carbonate, barium titanate, and others. Numerous factors contribute to the properties of particulate-filled denture base, including the type of filler, type of matrix, filler-matrix interaction, filler volume fraction, filler-filler interaction, voids, and defects. It has been observed by Harper et al. that smaller particle size yields better properties enhancement than larger particle size. Geometrically balanced particles, such as spherical glass beads, produce isotropic composites, while platelet and angular-shaped particles not only introduce anisotropy to the mechanical properties but also increase the viscosity of the melt [16].

The composite function employs a continuous phase matrix that serves the purpose of retaining the particulate filler while also providing it with a protective enclosure against both mechanical and chemical damage. Additionally, the matrix acts as a medium for overall stress distribution, allowing for applied loads to be passed on to the filler. It is crucial that the matrix possess the ability to distribute the particulate filler evenly in order to prevent agglomeration.

The mechanical and chemical properties of the composites, as well as their suitability for high temperature environments, are largely determined by the type of matrix utilized. The interaction between the filler and matrix occurs at the interface, which is a small region located between the contact surfaces of the two materials. This interaction plays a critical role in determining the extent to which the load is shared between the matrix and the filler. An effective interface is essential for the transfer of stress from the matrix to the filler, which possesses superior rigidity and strength. This mechanism allows for the reinforcement of the overall composites and thus enables them to endure higher levels of applied stress, resulting in improved properties. The interaction between filler and matrix, particularly in the case of mineral fillers such as hydroxyapatite and alumina with non-polar organic matrices, can be further improved with the use of coupling agents, typically silane coupling agents [17].

The silane coupling agent is comprised of two distinct components, each of which exhibits a strong affinity toward either the filler or the matrix. As a result, it functions as a bridge of sorts that enhances the interaction between the filler and matrix through the formation of a chemical bond between the two phases, as opposed to relying solely on a mechanical interlock [18].

Debnath et al. [19] investigated methacrylic resin-based dental composites treated with silane coupling agent to provide the interfacial phase that holds together the organic polymer matrix with the reinforcing inorganic phase. In this study, fiber pullout tests were used to measure the interfacial bond strength at the fiber-matrix interface. Glass fibers (approximately 30 μm diameter, 8 cm length, MoSci) were silanated using various concentrations (1, 5, and 10%) of either 3-methacryloxypropyl-trimethoxysilane (MPS) or glycidoxypropyl trimethoxy silane (GPS) in acetone (99.8%). Rubber (poly (butadiene/acrylonitrile), amine terminated, (Mw 5500) molecules were also attached to the fiber surface via GPS molecules. A positive correlation was found between the amount of silane on the filler surface and the property loss after soaking. Rubber treatment provided improvement in interfacial strength. 5% MPS samples had the highest strength both in soaked as well as unsoaked samples.

The filler volume fraction, also known as the filler content, plays a crucial role in determining the properties of a composite material. Typically, as the amount of filler increases, the modulus also increases, but this is accompanied by a greater brittleness in the material. The reason for this is that as more filler is added, the polymer content decreases [20]. In order to achieve the maximum loading of filler while maintaining the desired tensile strength and toughness of the polymer, it is essential that the filler is evenly distributed and that the interface between the filler and matrix is of high quality. Furthermore, as the amount of filler increases, it becomes increasingly important to consider the interactions between the individual filler particles [21].

The filler-filler interaction deals with the affinity of fillers toward each other and toward composite matrix. When the filler-filler interaction is stronger than the filler-matrix interaction, it leads to the clustering of fillers in a particular region. This, in turn, acts as a site of stress concentration which can result in premature failure or cracking. To mitigate this issue, the use of dispersing agents and effective mechanical mixing can be employed to decrease the filler-filler interaction. Additionally, voids and defects caused by the presence of moisture-containing fillers or during processing also have a significant impact on the properties of composite materials. In fact, they exhibit an effect that is equivalent to filler agglomeration, serving as a source of stress concentration and a site for crack initiation, ultimately leading to premature failure, as noted by Atkins and Mai [22].

3.1 Fibers

The filled of acrylic resin with fibers has been documented as a means of enhancing the flexural and impact strength, also to the fatigue resistance of the resin [23]. Numerous investigations have been carried out utilizing various kinds of fibers, including but not limited to nylon, polyethylene, polyamide fiber, and glass fiber, which are widely used owing to its biocompatibility and exceptional esthetic and mechanical characters [24].

3.1.1 Glass fiber

The utilization of glass fiber as a reinforcing agent has been discovered to produce a significant enhancement in the flexural strength, impact strength, fracture toughness, and Vickers hardness of acrylic resin, as evidenced by previous studies [25]. Moreover, it has been observed that deformation of the denture base is reduced to less than 1%. Researchers have found that the manner in which the glass fiber interacts with the denture base affects its properties. In particular, it has been reported that positioning the glass fiber in close proximity to the surface of the denture base leads to an improvement in flexural strength, fracture toughness, and flexural modulus. Conversely, placement of the glass fiber in neutral stress areas only enhances flexural toughness, while placement in the compressive side results in an increase in surface flexural modulus [26].

On the other hand, the findings of a study indicate that the impregnation of glass fiber into acrylic resin does not have an impact on its linear dimensional stability [27]. Additionally, the use of preimpregnated and silane-treated glass fiber, specifically with 3-(Trimethoxysilyl) propyl methacrylate (TMSPM), has been shown to increase both flexural and impact strength of the acrylic resin [28]. Furthermore, the introduction of silanized glass fiber to heat-cured and light-cured resins has been deemed biocompatible. Notably, the utilization of fiber-reinforced nanopigmented PMMA has been found to reduce porosity and *Candida albicans* adherence [29].

3.1.2 Polyamide fiber

Polyamide fibers, including both Nylon and Aramid fibers, were used to reinforce denture base. Research has shown that Aramid fiber reinforcement enhances the biocompatibility of the resin, while simultaneously increasing its flexural strength and modulus [30]. Nevertheless, it is worth noting that an increase in fiber concentration can lead to a decrease in the resin's hardness, which is considered a disadvantage. Additionally, the yellow color of the Aramid fiber is also regarded as a drawback [31]. On the other hand, Nylon has been found to improve the fracture resistance of PMMA due to its high resistance to continual stress. As a result, incorporating Nylon fiber into PMMA has been shown to increase its structural elasticity [32].

3.1.3 Polyethylene and polypropylene fibers

The incorporation of polyethylene fiber into PMMA resulted in a significant increase in impact strength, with even greater improvements observed through the application of fiber surface treatment, as previously noted in studies [33]. In contrast, while woven polyethylene fiber reinforcement has been shown to enhance the elastic modulus and toughness of PMMA, the practicality of fiber etching, preparation, and positioning has been reported to be difficult [34]. The use of polypropylene fiber, with surface treatment leading to further enhancements in impact strength [35]. In fact, plasma-treated polypropylene fibers have been found to provide the highest impact strength, offering a viable option for strengthening acrylic resin and reducing the likelihood of fracturing. Incorporating silanized polypropylene fiber into heat-cured PMMA resin has also been shown to significantly improve transverse, tensile, and impact strengths, although it should be noted that wear resistance may be negatively impacted [36].

3.1.4 Natural fibers

Two natural fibers, namely oil palm empty fruit bunch (OPEFB) and ramie fiber, have been utilized to reinforce denture base resins. The incorporation of OPEFB has led to a significant increase in the flexural strength and flexural modulus of acrylic resin, as evidenced by previous research [37]. Short ramie fiber, on the other hand, has been observed to increase the flexural modulus of acrylic resin relative to conventional PMMA. However, the flexural strength has decreased due to weak interfacial bonding between the filler and matrix. It should be noted that the long form of ramie fiber poses a disadvantage, as it necessitates additional work, such as cutting and preparation [38].

3.1.5 Hybrid reinforcement

The idea to reinforce PMMA with a variety of fibers was initially introduced by Vallittu [39]. This combination could include varied types of fibers, metal oxides, ceramics, and fibers with metal oxides or ceramic materials. The integration of hybrid fiber reinforcement has effectively increased the flexural strength and toughness of the reinforced acrylic resin. Similar results were noted through the inclusion of metal oxides and ceramics, specifically NPs, in PMMA. Moreover, this method provides improved surface roughness, tensile strength, flexural modulus, hardness, thermal conductivity, radiopacity, and reduced shrinkage. Additionally, it exhibits antibacterial properties without any cytotoxicity. A combination of fibers and other fillers has also resulted in an elevation of impact strength, hardness, surface roughness, and thermal conductivity, as well as compressive and fatigue strengths [40–43].

3.2 Fillers

Numerous investigations have demonstrated that the utilization of fillers amplifies the potency of denture base resin and markedly ameliorates its characteristics. The addition of nanofillers has been recommended as a means to augment the properties of PMMA. Nanofillers, owing to their elevated surface area, small dimensions, and uniform distribution, have been shown to enhance the thermal properties of PMMA and heighten its thermal stability in comparison to pure PMMA. The characteristics of the resin, which is reinforced by nanofillers, are contingent upon the magnitude, morphology, category, and concentration of the supplementary particles [44–47].

3.2.1 Metal oxides

Several investigations have indicated that the augmentation of PMMA with metal oxides has led to enhancements in both the physical and mechanical properties of the material, as well as the tactile sensations experienced by patients in response to hot and cold stimuli [48]. Consequently, the addition of metal fillers to denture base resin was expected to result in improved food sensation and healthier oral mucosa. Nevertheless, certain researchers have noted that the incorporation of metal oxides into acrylic resin has been observed to have a deleterious impact on the strength of the denture base, owing to stress concentration in the vicinity of the embedded metal particles and their weak adhesion to the polymer. Several techniques, including sand-blasting, silanization, and metal adhesive resins, have been recommended to enhance the bond between the acrylic resin and metal surface [49, 50].

3.2.2 Alumina (Al_2O_3)

The incorporation of alumina particles into acrylic resin has been found to have a positive impact on the properties of denture base, as reported previously [51]. Furthermore, the addition of alumina powder to acrylic resin has been shown to enhance its thermal conductivity and mechanical properties, according to previous research [52]. Additionally, the reinforcement of PMMA with Al_2O_3 has been found to increase the flexural strength, impact strength, tensile strength, compressive strength, and surface hardness of the resin. Moreover, the inclusion of aluminum in PMMA has been found to significantly reduce warpage. However, some studies have reported that the addition of aluminum decreases both the impact and tensile strength of PMMA. It has also been observed that the flexural properties of acrylic resin can be improved by treating Al_2O_3 particles with a coupling agent. Similarly, the treatment of aluminum particles with silane has been found to significantly increase the compressive, tensile, and flexural strength as well as the wear resistance of reinforced denture base resin, as reported in several studies [53–55].

The impact of alumina reinforced denture resin on surface roughness and water sorption has been investigated. One study observed no significant changes in these properties. However, another study found that the addition of Al_2O_3 resulted in a decrease in water sorption and solubility, while yet another study reported an increase in water sorption [56]. Additionally, the thermal stability of PMMA was found to increase upon the addition of Al_2O_3 nanoparticles. The thermal properties and flexural strength of acrylic resin were also shown to improve with the addition of silanized Al_2O_3 NPs, while water sorption and solubility decreased. Finally, biocompatibility was demonstrated when alumina NPs were added to both microwave-treated and untreated PMMA powder in a different study [57, 58].

The utilization of alumina-reinforced PMMA is hindered by the occurrence of resin discoloration, thereby restricting its application to non-visible areas. While the introduction of Al_2O_3 into PMMA resulted in a considerable enhancement of thermal conductivity, the flexural strength values of PMMA remained unaltered to a significant extent [59, 60].

3.2.3 Zirconia (ZrO_2)

The inclusion of zirconia (ZrO_2) fillers into PMMA resulted in a notable increase in its flexural strength, as reported by various studies [61, 62]. However, it was also observed that there was a slight reduction in the flexural strength, which could be attributed to the clustering of particles within the resin, leading to material weakness. Furthermore, the incorporation of ZrO_2 into PMMA led to a significant improvement in the impact strength, fracture toughness, and hardness, as documented in one study. Nonetheless, one study found that the impact strength and surface hardness of zirconia-reinforced resin did not increase significantly compared to unreinforced PMMA. In fact, a decrease in both impact strength and surface hardness was reported in some cases. It is important to note that the addition of ZrO_2 had a significant impact on the thermal conductivity of PMMA, which increased considerably. However, studies have yielded varying results with respect to the effect of ZrO_2 on the water sorption and solubility of PMMA. While some studies suggest that adding ZrO_2 led to a significant decrease in the water sorption and solubility of PMMA, other studies found an insignificant difference in water solubility and an increase in water sorption within the limit of ADA specifications [63, 64].

The inclusion of zirconia nanoparticles has been proposed as a means to enhance the mechanical properties of PMMA. The addition of zirconia nanoparticles to PMMA has been shown to increase its impact strength, flexural strength, compressive strength, fatigue strength, fracture toughness, and hardness. Furthermore, it has been suggested that zirconia nanoparticles may have antifungal properties and could potentially serve as a preventive measure for patients who are susceptible to fungal infections. However, one study has reported a negligible increase in the hardness of nano-ZrO_2/PMMA, and no significant alteration in its surface roughness [65–67].

The impact of the inclusion of ZrO_2 nanoparticles (NPs) on the color properties of PMMA was not found to possess any significant color alterations. To enhance the bond strength between ZrO_2 NPs and PMMA, a silane coupling agent was employed, resulting in an increase in the acrylic resin's flexural strength and impact strength; however, its tensile strength was not enhanced. Nonetheless, a study discovered that the incorporation of silanized ZrO_2NPs improved the tensile strength and fatigue strength of PMMA. Furthermore, the addition of silanized ZrO_2 NPs to acrylic resin resulted in a significant increase in hardness and a slight increase in surface roughness, while apparent porosity, water sorption, and solubility decreased. Additionally, zirconia nanotubes were found to exhibit a superior reinforcing effect compared to zirconia NPs. However, surface treatment would decrease the reinforcing effect of ZrO_2 nanotubes compared to ZrO_2 NPs. Specifically, flexural strength was optimized when 2 wt% untreated ZrO_2 nanotubes were incorporated into PMMA [68–70].

3.2.4 Hydroxyapatite (HA)

The utilization of bio-ceramic systems based in HA has proven to be a significant category of bioactive materials that can effectively promote bone regeneration and consequently facilitate a robust interface fixation between host tissues and medical or dental devices. The incorporation of HA can substantially improve the properties of denture base materials, particularly in terms of their radiopaque nature. Research has demonstrated that the addition of 5 and 10% HA that has been treated with γ-MPS significantly enhances the flexural, flexural toughness, tensile strength, and hardness of PMMA denture base resin. Furthermore, it has been observed that the radiopacity of denture base material is also elevated [9, 10, 16, 17].

The introduction of HA fillers to PMMA results in superior mechanical properties, including an increase in flexural strength and flexural modulus of PMMA. This is primarily due to the enhanced interfacial interaction between the HA filler and the PMMA matrix that is brought about by the treatment with γ-MPS. However, the immersion of PMMA in water has been found to cause a reduction in the flexural properties due to water's plasticizing effect, which weakens the bonding between the HA filler and the PMMA matrix. In contrast, the addition of HA NPs has been shown to increase both the fatigue and compression strength of PMMA resin in comparison with pure PMMA, in addition to inducing a significant increase in thermal conductivity [11, 12].

3.2.5 Titanium (TiO_2)

Numerous investigations have been conducted to examine the impact of the inclusion of TiO_2 on the attributes of PMMA. It has been determined that the introduction of TiO_2 particles may enhance the flexural strength, fracture toughness, and hardness of PMMA as well as its thermal conductivity. Furthermore, the incorporation of TiO_2 into PMMA has been shown to cause a noteworthy increase in impact strength, while simultaneously leading to a significant reduction in water sorption and solubility [71].

In contrast, certain investigations have indicated that the incorporation of TiO_2 into PMMA does not enhance its flexure strength due to the clustering of particles within the resin, thereby compromising its structural integrity. However, research has demonstrated that the introduction of TiO_2 nanoparticles into PMMA can influence its thermal properties (such as a reduction in thermal expansion coefficient and contraction) and mechanical stability (with a decrease in E-modulus), although it may result in a reduction in flexural strength and toughness.

To optimize the properties of PMMA composite, it is crucial to ensure strong adhesion between the resin matrix and filler particles, which can be achieved by employing a titanium coupling agent to reinforce titanium-reinforced PMMA. Furthermore, the addition of silanized TiO_2 nanoparticles to PMMA has been observed to improve its impact strength, transverse strength, and surface hardness, while reducing water sorption and solubility. However, it also increased surface roughness after adding 3 wt% of silanized TiO_2 nanoparticles to acrylic resin [11, 72]. Additionally, the incorporation of apatite-coated titanium dioxide and fluoridated apatite-coated titanium dioxide into PMMA, followed by ultraviolet irradiation, has been found to effectively prevent candida adhesion due to their antifungal properties, thereby promoting appropriate denture hygiene. However, the addition of $BaTiO_3$ as a radiopacifier to PMMA resulted in a slight decline in fracture toughness properties. Although PMMA/$BaTiO_3$ composite material has demonstrated thermal stability, its increased density could compromise denture retention [11].

3.2.6 Silicon dioxide (SiO_2)

Numerous investigations have been carried out to examine the impact of the addition of SiO_2 on the properties of PMMA. It has been determined that the mechanical and thermal properties of PMMA can be improved by incorporating SiO_2 nanoparticles (NPs). The introduction of SiO_2 NPs has led to an enhancement in both the transverse and impact strength of PMMA. Additionally, surface hardness has been observed to increase with a higher concentration of SiO_2 NPs. However, it has been discovered that a low concentration of SiO_2 NPs can lead to an improvement in both hardness and fracture toughness. Conversely, an increase in SiO_2 NPs content results in agglomeration and crack propagation, which can reduce both hardness and fracture toughness [73, 74].

The inclusion of surface-treated SiO_2 has been found to enhance the flexural strength of PMMA, albeit it does not affect the hardness. In contrast, a recent study has revealed that silica NPs have an adverse effect on the flexural strength of PMMA. The reinforcement of acrylic resin with glass flakes, which are silica-based fillers, has been found to improve its fracture toughness. Furthermore, the use of silane coupling has resulted in further enhancement of the resin's properties. Micas, a group of lamellar silicate minerals, have also been proposed as a means of improving the properties of resin. These minerals are characterized by their high aspect ratio and have been observed to enhance the mechanical, thermal, and dimensional properties of PMMA. The incorporation of mica has been found to increase the hardness of acrylic resin, while its flexural strength has been reduced due to the weak bond between mica and the acrylic resin [75–77].

The incorporation of fluoride glass fillers into PMMA has been observed to reduce microbial adhesion, albeit with a slight increase in the surface roughness of the denture base resin. This was documented in Refs [78]. Additionally, the utilization of nanoclay as an additive in composite and acrylic polymers has been noted to enhance their properties. It was found that the introduction of nanoclay particles into PMMA led to an improvement in its thermal conductivity, albeit at the expense of its flexural strength, as reported in Ref. Furthermore, the placement of silicon carbide filler powders in the palatal region of dentures has been shown to enhance the thermal conductivity of PMMA without compromising its strength or increasing its weight. This was detailed in Ref. [79].

3.2.7 Polyetheretherketone (PEEK)

Polyetheretherketone (PEEK) is a semi-crystalline engineering plastic that exhibits its remarkable mechanical and thermal properties. With its impressive advantages, including its lightweight nature, non-toxicity, corrosion resistance, and low modulus closely resembling that of natural bone, PEEK has emerged as a highly promising clinical implant for orthopedic applications [80, 81].

Recently, PEEK has been introduced to enhance the general mechanical performance of the PMMA resin base. The PMMA resin has been combined with TiO_2 and PEEK, leading to a significant improvement in both the average bending strength and the flexural modulus [82]. In the realm of dental implant applications, Chen et al. [83] have found PEEK compounds to be promising restorative materials. Moreover, a recent study Schwitalla et al. [84] has demonstrated that the mechanical properties of PEEK were unaffected by artificial saliva solution with different pH values over a period of 30 days at 25°C. There are some studies that suggest PEEK as a potential restorative material in the oral cavity [85, 86].

Chen et al. [83] developed a practical and convenient protocol for light-curing resin utilized in the 3D industry. This protocol enhances the antibacterial and mechanical properties of PMMA resin through the combination of nanofillers of surface-modified TiO_2 and micro-fillers of PEEK. The study's findings demonstrated that PMMA composite resins reinforced with TiO_2–1%-PEEK-1% exhibited the most optimized properties. The researchers concluded that the incorporation of 1% of TiO_2 would be an effective amount to enhance both the mechanical and antibacterial properties of PMMA composite resin. In addition, the PMMA (TiO_2–1%-PEEK-1%) composite resin's printed model presented a smooth surface and precise resolution. This indicates that the functional dental restoration material would be a suitable light-curing resin in the 3D industry [83].

3.2.8 Silver (Ag)

Several studies have reported that the inclusion of silver nanoparticles (AgNPs) in denture base acrylic resin exhibits antifungal properties. This effect is particularly noticeable at high concentrations and has been shown to act as a latent antifungal material, with low-releasing Ag^+ [84–87]. Conversely, Wady et al. [88] found that the incorporation of silver NPs in PMMA did not impact the adhesion of *C. albicans* and biofilm accumulation. The addition of silver to PMMA is known to possess antimicrobial properties, which can reduce microbial adhesion and colonization. As such, it may be beneficial for immune-compromised and geriatric patients. Furthermore, PMMA reinforced with silver has been shown to increase flexural and fatigue strength, as well as improve thermal conductivity. Another study revealed that the incorporation of 0.5% antimicrobial silver-zinc zeolite in heat-cured acrylic resin did not affect its impact and transverse strength, surface hardness, or surface roughness. However, it did result in a significant decrease in water sorption and an increase in water solubility. It has been suggested that the mechanical properties of denture base resin may be negatively affected by the addition of silver, depending on its percentage [88, 89].

Incorporating silane-treated Ag particles significantly increased the compressive strength of PMMA. Also, addition of 10 and 20 wt% silane-treated silver fillers enhanced the tensile and flexural strength of PMMA. The inclusion of silane-treated silver particles demonstrated a noteworthy increase in the compressive strength of PMMA. Furthermore, when 10 and 20 wt% silane-treated silver fillers were added, both the tensile and flexural strength of PMMA were enhanced. The introduction of silver powder to PMMA also led to a significant increase in thermal conductivity, while the flexural strength values of PMMA remained unaltered. The physical and mechanical properties of PMMA were improved by the incorporation of silver nanoparticles (NPs), including increased thermal conductivity and compressive strength [90].

Hence, the application of Ag NPs is recommended in the palatal region of maxillary acrylic resin dentures. Additionally, it has been determined that PMMA-silver NPs do not exhibit cytotoxicity. However, the tensile strength of PMMA did not undergo significant changes after the inclusion of 0.2% Ag NPs in comparison with unmodified PMMA. Nevertheless, a significant decrease in tensile strength was observed after the incorporation of 2% Ag NPs. Moreover, PMMA-Ag NPs have been reported to exhibit poor color stability. The addition of AgNPs to acrylic denture base material can enhance its viscoelastic properties [91].

The potential benefits of incorporating nano-gold (Au), platinum (Pt), and palladium (Pd) into PMMA denture base have been suggested in recent studies. However, the available literature on the effects of adding nano-gold to PMMA remains limited. Encouragingly, it has been observed that the inclusion of Au NPs can significantly enhance the flexural strength and thermal conductivity of PMMA, resulting in nearly double the value of pure PMMA and potentially increasing patient satisfaction. Additionally, the addition of Pt NPs may improve the mechanical properties of PMMA and provide an antimicrobial effect [92].

The results of the investigation revealed that the utilization of Pt led to a notable increase in the bending deflection of PMMA. Furthermore, it was observed that palladium had a positive impact on the bending strength of the material, in contrast to silver and gold, which both exhibited the lowest level of bending strength. Additionally, the incorporation of gold and palladium proved to enhance the Vickers hardness of PMMA, whereas the introduction of platinum was shown to have a decreasing effect on this property [93].

The halloysite nanotube, a naturally occurring silica-based mineral, was initially introduced by Abdallah [94] in 2016 as a means to enhance the properties of PMMA. It was observed that the addition of halloysite nanotube in small proportions led to an increase in the hardness of PMMA, however, there was no significant improvement in the flexural strength and Young's modulus. The use of carbon family fillers, specifically carbon fillers, to reinforce PMMA, is not a common practice due to issues such as biological complications, suboptimal esthetics, and challenges in handling and polishing. However, nano-carbon has emerged as a prominent sector of nanotechnology in recent times [92].

3.2.9 Nano-carbon

The introduction of carbon nanotubes at a rate of 1% into PMMA led to a significant increase in both the impact strength and flexural strength of the resin, albeit at the cost of decreased hardness, according to one study. Another study found that the addition of 1.5% single-walled carbon nanotubes had a significant effect on the impact and transverse strength of PMMA, yet led to a noticeable reduction in surface hardness. In contrast, a separate study revealed that the addition of single-walled carbon nanotubes had an insignificant effect on the flexural strength of PMMA. Furthermore, the incorporation of 0.5 and 1% multiple-wall carbon nanotubes (MWCNTs) into PMMA resulted in an improvement in both the flexural strength and resilience of the resin, but with higher concentrations of MWCNTs, the fatigue resistance was seen to decrease [93].

3.2.10 Nano-diamonds

The exceptional characteristics of nano-diamonds, specifically their high level of hardness and thermal conductivity, have led researchers to explore their potential for enhancing the mechanical properties of PMMA. The incorporation of NDs into PMMA resulted in a significant increase in impact strength, as well as an improvement in fracture toughness, albeit only at the lowest concentration of NDs. Additionally, the scratch resistance of PMMA was shown to be enhanced through the use of heat-treated NDs. However, the agglomeration of the nanoparticles was identified as a primary drawback, as it could potentially serve as a site for stress concentration [95].

4. Advanced perspective dental prosthesis

The employment of digital dentistry technology has emerged as the prevailing trend in dental prosthetics across the globe in contemporary times. The advent of digital three-dimensional (3D) printing technology has significantly enhanced the diagnostic rate and demonstrated remarkable potential in the realm of personalized medicine. In comparison to the conventional manufacturing process, 3D-printed prostheses boast shorter production cycles and higher precision, thereby optimizing the comfort of denture patients. Presently, approximately 75% of 3D printing dental applications utilize light-curing technology, wherein light-curing resins are extensively used as fillers and restorative materials in stomatology. PMMA is a widely used commercial light-curing resin in the 3D printing industry owing to its low odor, low irritancy, good flexibility, and cost-effectiveness. However, the inherent limitations of PMMA, including substantial shrinkage rate during light-curing, brittleness, poor mechanical properties, and low antibacterial activity, among others, have restricted its widespread clinical application. Hence, further research and development are imperative to enhance the existing properties of 3D printing denture base materials [96, 97].

5. Conclusion

Although PMMA has been utilized for constructing denture bases and has become the preferred material for such fabrication, it exhibits low fracture resistance, specifically under fatigue failure within the oral cavity and impact failure outside of it. Consequently, various reinforcement agents, such as fibers or filler particles in micro and nano scales, have been investigated to enhance the properties of denture base materials. This has resulted in the expanded use of dental composites in numerous applications, which in turn has spurred the demand for continued research and improvement to enhance their properties and performance. One promising approach involves employing a nanofiller modified with a silane coupling agent to improve the dispersibility of fillers in a polymer, thereby enhancing the mechanical properties of the composite resin. The future of manufacturing applications in three-dimensional (3D) printing and CAD/CAM technology of denture base resins with improved properties will necessitate the development of materials suitable for 3D printing technology and denture base applications.

Conflict of interest

The author declares no conflict of interest.

Author details

Saied H. Mohamed
Faculty of Dentistry, Prosthodontics Department, University of Benghazi, Libya

*Address all correspondence to: saied.alabidi@uob.edu.ly

References

[1] Anusavice KJ, Shen C, Rawls R. Ch. 19. In: Phillips' Science of Dental Materials. Library of Congress Cataloging-in-Publication Data or Control Number Mosby. 12th ed. Printed in China; 2013. pp. 465-466

[2] Ferracane JL. Ch. 2. In: Material in Dentistry Principles and Applications. 2nd ed. Philadelphia, USA: J. B. Lippincott Williams & Wilkins; 2001. pp. 10-17

[3] John J, Gandahar SA, Shah I. Flexural strength of heat-polymerized poly methyl methyl methacrylate denture resin reinforced with glass, aramid, or nylon fibers. The Journal of Prosthetic Dentistry. 2001;**86**:424-427

[4] Rudigier J, Dreaner K, Grunert A, Ritter G. Effects of adding X-ray contrast materials to bone cements. J. Acts Traumat. 1977;7:35-38

[5] Davy KWM, Anseau MR, Berry C. Iodinated methacrylate copolymers as X-ray opaque denture base acrylics. Journal of Dentistry. 1997;**25**:499-505

[6] Deb SV, BT. The effect of cross-linking agents on acrylic bone cements containing radiopacifiers. Journal of Biomaterials. 2001;**22**:2177-2181

[7] Van Hooy-Corstjens CSJ, Govaert LE, Spoelstra AB, et al. Mechanical properties of a new acrylic radiopaque iodine-containing bone cement. Journal of Biomaterials. 2004;**25**:2657-2666

[8] Lewis GA. Properties of acrylic bone cement; state of the art review. Journal of Biomedical Materials Research Part B: Applied Biomaterials. 1997;**38**:155-182

[9] Abboud M, Vol S, Duguet E, Fontanille M. PMMA-based composite materials with reactive ceramic filler, part III. Radiopacifying particle-reinforced bone cements. Journal of Materials Science. Materials in Medicine. 2000;**11**:295-300

[10] Mohamed SH. Physical, Mechanical and Biological Properties of PMMA Denture Base Material Filled with Ceramic Filler [Thesis]. Penang, Malaysia: USM; Polymeric Engineer, University Science Malaysia; 2006

[11] Elshereksi NW, Mohamed SH, Arifin Z, Mohd Ishak ZA. Effect of filler incorporation on the fracture toughness properties of denture base poly (methyl methacrylate). Journal of Physical Science. 2009;**20**(2):1-12

[12] Mohamed SH, Arifin Z, Mohd Ishak ZA. The effect of physical mixing on mechanical properties of hydroxyapatite filled poly (methyl methacrylate). Journal of the Institute of Materials Malaysia (JIMM). 2003:**4**(2):10-18

[13] Yee A. Impact resistance.In. In: Mark HF, editor. Encyclopedia of Polymer Science and Technology. 2nd ed. Vol. 8. New York: Wiley; 1987. pp. 36-68

[14] Cho K, Yang JHP, CE. The effect of rubber particle size on toughening behaviour of rubber-modified poly (methyl methacrylate) with different test methods. Journal of Polymer. 1998;**14**:3073-3081

[15] Zappini G, Kammann A, Wachter W. Comparison of fracture tests of denture base materials. The Journal of Prosthetic Dentistry. 2003;**90**:578-585

[16] Harper EJ, Braden M, Bonfield W. Mechanical properties of hydroxyapatite

reinforced poly (ethylmethacrylate) bone cement after immersion in a physiological solution: Influence of a silane coupling agent. Journal of Materials Science: Materials in Medicine. 2000;**11**:491-497

[17] Wang M, Bonfield W. Chemically coupled hydroxyapatite-polyethylene composites; structure and properties. Journal of Biomaterials. 2001;**22**:1311-1320

[18] Fu Q, Wang G, Liu C. Polyethylene toughened by $CaCO_3$ particles, the interface behaviour and fracture mechanism in high density polyethylene/ CaCO3 blends. Journal of Polymer. 1995;**36**:2387-2401

[19] Debnath S, Wunder SL, JI MC, Baran GR. Silane treatment effects on glass/resin interfacial shear strengths. International Journal of Dental Materials. 2003;**19**:441-448

[20] Silva ALN, Rocha MCG, Moraes MAR, CAR V, Coutinho FMB. Mechanical and rheological properties of composites based on polyolefin and mineral additives. Journal of Polymer Testing. 2002;**21**:57-60

[21] Rusu M, Sofian N, Rusu D. Mechanical and thermal properties of zinc powder filled high density polyethylene composites. Journal of Polymer testing. 2001;**20**:409-417

[22] Atkins AG, Mai YW. Elastic and Plastic Fracture Metals, Polymers Ceramics, Biological Materials. Chichester: Ellis Horwood Limited; 1985

[23] Alla R, Sajjan S, Alluri V, Ginjupalli K, Padhya NU. Influence of fiber reinforcement on the properties of denture base resins. Journal of Biomaterials and Nanobiotechnology. 2013;**4**:91-97

[24] Tacir IH, Kama JD, Zortuk M, Eskimez S. Flexural properties of glass fiber reinforced acrylic resin polymers. Australian Dental Journal. 2006;**51**:52-56

[25] Moreno MV, Acosta-Torres LS, Barcel Osantana FH, Vanegas-Lanc RD, Plata-Rodrı'guez ME, Casta VM. Fiber-reinforced nano-pigmented poly (methyl methacrylate) as improved denture base. Journal of Applied Polymer Science. 2012;**126**:289-296

[26] Sang-Hui YU, Yoon LE, Seunghan OH, Hye-Won CH, Yutaka OD, Ji-Myung BA. Reinforcing effects of different fibers on denture base resin based on the fiber type, concentration, and combination. Dental Materials Journal. 2012;**3**:1039-1046

[27] Farina AP, Cecchin D, Soares RG, et al. Evaluation of vickers hardness of different types of acrylic denture base resins with and without glass fiber reinforcement. Gerodontology. 2012;**29**:155-160

[28] Hamouda IM, Beyari MM. Addition of glass fibers and titanium dioxide nanoparticles to the acrylic resin denture base material: Comparative study with the conventional and high impact types. Oral Health and Dental Management. 2014;**13**:107-112

[29] Singh K, Sharma SK, Negi P, Kumar M, Rajpurohit D, Khobre P. Comparative evaluation of flexural strength of heat polymerized denture base resins after reinforcement with glass fibers and nylon fibers: An in vitro study. Advances in Human Biology. 2016;**6**:91-94

[30] Agha H, Flinton R, Vaidyanathan T. Optimization of fracture resistance and stiffness of heat-polymerized high impact acrylic resin with localized e-glass fiber reinforcement at different

stress points. Journal of Prosthodontics. 2016;**25**(8):647-655

[31] Fonseca RB, Favarão IN, Kasuya VB, Abrão M, Da Luz NFM, Naves LZ. Influence of glass fiber wt% and silanization on mechanical flexural strength of reinforced acrylics. Journal of Materials Science and Chemical Engineering. 2014;**2**:11-15

[32] Yu SH, Ahn DH, Park JS, et al. Comparison of denture base resin reinforced with polyaromatic polyamide fibers of different orientations. Dental Materials Journal. 2013;**32**:332-340

[33] Chen SY, Liang WM, Yen PS. Reinforcement of acrylic denture base resin by incorporation of various fibers. Journal of Biomedical Materials Research. 2001;**58**:203-208

[34] Soygun K, Bolayir G, Boztug A. Mechanical and thermal properties of polyamide versus reinforced PMMA denture base materials. The Journal of Advanced Prosthodontics. 2013;**5**:153-160

[35] Uzun G, Hersek N, Tinçer T. Effect of five woven fiber reinforcements on the impact and transverse strength of a denture base resin. The Journal of Prosthetic Dentistry. 1999;**81**:616-620

[36] Ismaeel IJ, Alalwan HA, Mustafa MJ. The effect of the addition of silanated polypropylene fiber to polymethylmethacrylate denture base material on some of its mechanical properties. Journal of Baghdad College of Dentistry. 2015;**27**:40-47

[37] John J, Ann Mani S, Palaniswamy K, Ramanathan A, Razak AA. Flexural properties of poly (methyl methacrylate) resin reinforced with oil palm empty fruit bunch fibers: A preliminary finding. Journal of Prosthodontics. 2015;**24**:233-238

[38] Xu J, Li Y, Yu T, Cong L. Reinforcement of denture base resin with short vegetable fiber. Dental Materials. 2013;**29**:1273-1279

[39] Vallittu PK, Narva K. Impact strength of a modified continuous glass fiber polymethylmethacrylate. The International Journal of Prosthodontics. 1997;**10**:142-148

[40] Safarabadia M, Khansarib NM, Rezaeic A. An experimental investigation of HA/AL2 O3 nanoparticles on mechanical properties of restoration materials. Engineering Solid Mechanics. 2014;**2**:173-182

[41] Han Z, Zhu B, Chen R, Huang Z, Zhu C, Zhang X. Effect of silver supported materials on the mechanical and antibacterial properties of reinforced acrylic resin composites. Materials and Design. 2015;**65**:1245-1252

[42] Aljafery MA, Basima MA. Effect of addition ZrO_2-Al_2 O_3 nanoparticles mixture on some properties and denture base adaptation of heat cured acrylic resin denture base material. Journal of Baghdad College of Dentistry. 2015;**27**:15-21

[43] Alhareb AO, Akil HM, Ahmad ZA. Mechanical properties of PMMA Denture Base reinforced by nitrile rubber particles with Al2O3/YSZ fillers. Procedia Manufacturing. 2015;**2**:301-306

[44] Muklif OR, Ismail IJ. Studying the effect of addition a composite of silanized Nano-Al_2 O_3 and plasma treated polypropylene fibers on some physical and mechanical properties of heat cured PMMA denture base material. Journal of Baghdad College of Dentistry. 2015;**27**:22-27

[45] Alhareb AO, Ahmad ZA. Effect of Al2 O3/ZrO2 reinforcement on the

mechanical properties of PMMA denture base. Journal of Reinforced Plastics and Composites. 2011;**30**:1-8

[46] Zhang XY, Zhang XJ, Huang ZL, Zhu BS, Chen RR. Hybrid effects of zirconia nanoparticles with aluminum borate whiskers on mechanical properties of denture base resin PMMA. Dental Materials Journal. 2014;**33**:141-146

[47] Salman TA, Khalaf HA. The influence of adding of modified ZrO2 - TiO2 nanoparticles on certain physical and mechanical properties of heat polymerized acrylic resin. Journal of Baghdad College of Dentistry. 2015;**27**:33-39

[48] Oei JD, Zhao WW, Chu L, et al. Antimicrobial acrylic materials with in situ generated silver nanoparticles. Journal of Biomedical Materials Research. 2012;**100**:409-415

[49] Yadav P, Mittal R, Sood VK, Garg R. Effect of incorporation of silane treated silver and aluminum microparticles on strength and thermal conductivity of PMMA. Journal of Prosthodontics. 2012;**21**:546-551

[50] Asar NV, Albayrak H, Korkmaz T, Turkyilmaz I. Influence of various metal oxides on mechanical and physical properties of heat-cured polymethylmethacrylate denture base resins. The Journal of Advanced Prosthodontics. 2013;**5**:241-247

[51] Sehajpal SB. Effect of metal fillers on some physical properties of acrylic resin. The Journal of Prosthetic Dentistry. 1989;**61**:746-751

[52] Safi IN. Evaluation the effect of nano-fillers (TiO2, AL2 O3, SiO2) addition on glass transition temperature, E-Moudulus and coefficient of thermal expansion of acrylic denture base material. Journal of Baghdad College of Dentistry. 2014;**26**:37-41

[53] Arora P, Singh SP, Arora V. Effect of alumina addition on properties of polymethylmethacrylate – A comprehensive review. International Journal of Biotech Trends and Technology. 2015;**9**:1-7

[54] Ellakwa AE, Morsy MA, El-Sheikh AM. Effect of aluminum oxide addition on the flexural strength and thermal diffusivity of heat-polymerized acrylic resin. Journal of Prosthodontics. 2008;**17**:439-444

[55] Vojdani M, Bagheri R, Khaledi AR. Effects of aluminum oxide addition on the flexural strength, surface hardness, and roughness of heat-polymerized acrylic resin. Journal of Dental Sciences. 2012;**7**:238-244

[56] Yadav NS, Elkawash H. Flexural strength of denture base resin reinforced with aluminum oxide and processed by different processing techniques. Journal of Advanced Medical and Dental Sciences Research. 2011;**2**:33-36

[57] Chaijareenont P, Takahashi H, Nishiyama N, Arksornnukit M. Effect of different amounts of 3-methacryloxypropyltrimethoxy silane on the flexural properties and wear resistance of alumina reinforced PMMA. Dental Materials Journal. 2012;**31**:623-628

[58] Arora N, Jain V, Chawla A, Mathur VP. Effect of addition of sapphire (aluminum oxide) or silver fillers on the flexural strength, thermal diffusivity and water sorption of heat-polymerized acrylic resins. International Journal of Prosthodontics and Restorative Dentistry. 2011;**1**:21-27

[59] Jasim BS, Ismail IJ. The effect of silanized alumina nano-fillers addition on

some physical and mechanical properties of heat cured polymethylmethacrylate denture base material. Journal of Baghdad College of Dentistry. 2014;**26**:18-23

[60] Abdulkareem MM, Hatim NA. Evaluation the biological effect of adding aluminum oxide, silver nanoparticles into microwave treated PMMA powder. International Journal of Enhanced Research In Science Technology & Engineering. 2015;**4**:172-178

[61] Asopa V, Suresh S, Khandelwal M, Sharma V, Asopa SS, Kairal LS. A comparative evaluation of properties of zirconia reinforced high impact acrylic resin with that of high impact acrylic resin. The Saudi Journal for Dental Research. 2015;**6**:146-151

[62] Ayad NM, Badawi MF, Fatah AA. Effect of reinforcement of high impact acrylic resin with zirconia on some physical and mechanical properties. Rev Clín Pesq Odontol. 2008;**4**:145-151

[63] Gad MM, Rahoma A, Al-Thobity AM, ArRejaie AS. Influence of incorporation of ZrO2 nanoparticles on the repair strength of PMMAdenture bases. International Journal of Nanomedicine. 2016;**11**:5633-5643

[64] Zhang XJ, Zhang XY, Zhu BS, Qian C. Effect of nano ZrO_2 on flexural strength and surface hardness of polymethylmethacrylate. Shanghai Kou Qiang Yi Xue. 2011;**20**:358-363

[65] Gad M, ArRejaie AS, Abdel-Halim MS, Rahoma A. The reinforcement effect of nano-zirconia on the transverse strength of repaired acrylic denture base. International Journal of Dentistry. 2016;**2016**:7094056

[66] Ahmed MA, Ebrahim MI. Effect of zirconium oxide nano-fillers addition on the flexural strength, fracture toughness, and hardness of heat-polymerized acrylic resin. World Journal of Nano Science and Engineering. 2014;**4**:50-57

[67] Cierech M, Kolenda A, Grudniak AM, et al. Significance of polymathyl methacrylate (PMMA) modification by zinc oxide nanoparticles for fungal biofilm formation. International Journal of Pharmaceutics. 2016;**510**(1):323-335

[68] Safi IN, Hassanen KA, Ali NA. Assessment of zirconium oxide nano fillers incorporation and silanation on impact, tensile strength and color alteration of heat polymerized acrylic resin. Journal of Baghdad College of Dentistry. 2012;**24**:36-42

[69] Hameed HK, Abdul RH. The effect of addition nano particle ZrO_2 on some properties of autoclave processed heat cures acrylic denture base material. Journal of Baghdad College of Dentistry. 2015;**27**:32-39

[70] Mohammed D, Mudhaffar M. Effect of modified zirconium oxide nano-fillers addition on some properties of heat cure acrylic denture base material. Journal of Baghdad College of Dentistry. 2012;**24**:1-7

[71] Wei Y, Wang X, Tang Q, Guo M, Zhao J. Reinforcement of denture base PMMA with ZrO2 nanotubes. Journal of the Mechanical Behavior of Biomedical Materials. 2014;**32**:192-197

[72] Alwan SA, Alameer SS. The effect of the addition of silanized Nano titania fillers on some physical and mechanical properties of heat cured acrylic denture base materials. Journal of Baghdad College of Dentistry. 2015;**27**:86-91

[73] Elshereksi NW, Mohamed SM, Arifin Z, Mohd Ishak ZA. Thermal characterization of poly (methyl

methacrylate) filled with barium titanate as denture base material. Journal of Physical Science. 2014;**25**:15-27

[74] Alnamel HA, Mudhaffer M. The effect of silicon dioxide Nano-fillers reinforcement on some properties of heat-cure polymethylmethacrylate denture base material. Journal of Baghdad College of Dentistry. 2014;**26**:32-36

[75] Balos S, Pilic B, Markovic D, Pavlicevic J, Luzanin O. PMMAnanocomposites with low silica addition. The Journal of Prosthetic Dentistry. 2014;**111**:327-334

[76] Franklin P, Wood DJ, Bubb NL. Reinforcement of poly (methyl methacrylate) denture base with glass flake. Dental Materials. 2005;**21**:365-370

[77] Ghaffari T, Barzegar A, Hamedi Rad F, Moslehifard E. Effect of nanoclay on thermal conductivity and flexural strength of PMMAacrylic resin. Journal of Dentistry (Shiraz). 2016;**17**(2):121-127

[78] Cevik P, Yildirim-Bicer AZ. The effect of silica and prepolymer nanoparticles on the mechanical properties of denture base acrylic resin. Journal of Prosthodontics. 2018;**27**(8):763-770 Epub 2016 Nov 29

[79] Al-Bakri IA, Harty D, Al-Omari WM, Swain MV, Chrzanowski W, Ellakwa A. Surface characteristics and microbial adherence ability of modified polymethylmethacrylate by fluoridated glass fillers. Australian Dental Journal. 2014;**59**(4):482-489

[80] Kul E, Aladağ Lİ, Yeşildal R. Evaluation of thermal conductivity and flexural strength properties of poly (methyl methacrylate denture) base material reinforced with different fillers. The Journal of Prosthetic Dentistry. 2016;**116**:803-810

[81] Brockett C, Carbone S, Abdelgaied A, Fisher J, Jennings L. Influence of contact pressure, cross-shear and counterface material on the wear of PEEK and CFR-PEEK for orthopaedic applications. Journal of the Mechanical Behavior of Biomedical Materials. 2016;**63**:10-16

[82] Trindade R, Albrektsson T, Galli S, Prgomet Z, Tengvall P, Wennerberg A. Bone immune response to materials, part I: Titanium, PEEK and copper in comparison to sham at 10 days in rabbit tibia. Journal of Clinical Medicine. 2018;**7**:526

[83] Chen SG, Yang JY, Jia YG, Lu B, Ren L. TiO2 and PEEK reinforced 3D printing PMMA composite resin for dental Denture Base applications. Nanomaterials. 2019;**9**:1049. DOI: 10.3390/nano9071049

[84] Schwitalla AD, Zimmermann T, Spintig T, Kallage I, Müller W-D. Fatigue limits of different PEEK materials for dental implants. Journal of the Mechanical Behavior of Biomedical Materials. 2017;**69**:163-168

[85] Gao S, Gao S, Xu B, Yu H. Effects of different pH-values on the Nanomechanical surface properties of PEEK and CFR-PEEK compared to dental resin-based materials. Materials. 2015;**8**:4751-4767

[86] Stawarczyk B, Beuer F, Wimmer T, Jahn D, Sener B, Roos M, et al. Polyetheretherketone—A suitable material for fixed dental prostheses? Journal of Biomedical Materials Research Part B: Applied Biomaterials. 2014;**101**:1209-1216

[87] Acosta-Torres LS, Mendieta I, Nuñez-Anita RE, Cajero-Juárez M, Castaño VM. Cytocompatible antifungal acrylic resin containing silver

nanoparticles for dentures. International Journal of Nanomedicine. 2012;**7**:1-10

[88] Wady AF, Machado AL, Zucolotto V, Zamperini CA, Berni E, Vergani CE. Evaluation of Candida albicans adhesion and biofilm formation on a denture base acrylic resin containing silver nanoparticles. Journal of Applied Microbiology. 2012;**112**:1163-1172

[89] Ghafari T, Hamedi-Rad F, Ezzati B. Does addition of silver nanoparticles to denture base resin increase its thermal conductivity? The Journal of Dental Sciences. 2014;**32**:139-144

[90] Ghaffari T, Hamedi-rad F, Ezzati B. In vitro comparison of compressive and tensile strengths of acrylic resins reinforced by silver nanoparticles at 2% and 0.2% concentrations. Journal of Dental Research Dental Clinics Dental Prospects. 2014;**8**:204-209

[91] Morsy MA, Al-Daous MA. Gold nanoparticles-PMMA composite for denture base: Synthesis, mechanical and thermal characteristics. AKU Journal of Science and Engineering. 2014;**14**:369-374

[92] Wang R, Kayacan R, Küçükeşmen C. Nanotubes/PMMAcomposite resins as denture base materials. In: Zhang M, Naik RR, Dai L, editors. Carbon Nanomaterials for Biomedical Applications. 1st ed. Berlin: Springer International Publishing; 2015. pp. 227-240

[93] Mahmood WS. The effect of incorporating carbon nanotubes on impact, transverse strength, hardness, and roughness to high impact denture base material. Journal of Baghdad College of Dentistry. 2015;**27**:96-99

[94] Abdallah RM. Evaluation of PMMA resin mechanical properties with incorporated halloysite nanotubes. The Journal of Advanced Prosthodontics. 2016;**8**:167-171

[95] Jamróz W, Szafraniec J, Kurek M, Jachowicz R. 3D printing in pharmaceutical and medical applications. Recent Achievements and Challenges in Pharmaceutical Research. 2018;**35**:176

[96] Hammesfahr PD, O'Connor MT, Wang X. Light-curing technology: Past, present, and future. The Compendium of Continuing Education in Dentistry. 2002;**23**:18-24

[97] Totu EE, Nechifor AC, Nechifor G, Aboul-Enein HY, Cristache CM. Poly(methyl methacrylate) with TiO_2 nanoparticles inclusion for stereolitographic complete denture manufacturing—The future in dental care for elderly edentulous patients? Journal of Dentistry. 2017;**59**:68-77

Chapter 7

Full-Arch Implant-Supported Restorations: Hybrid versus Monolithic Design

Ioan Achim Borsanu, Ralph-Alexandru Erdelyi, Laura Rusu, Sergiu Manuel Antonie and Emanuel Adrian Bratu

Abstract

The selection of materials for full-arch restorations remains a critical decision for clinicians, with ongoing debates surrounding the utilization of hybrid versus monolithic materials. This book chapter provides a comprehensive exploration of the considerations, challenges, and implications associated with these material choices. Beginning with an overview of historical and contemporary material landscapes, the chapter delves into the dynamic interplay between hybrid and monolithic materials, examining their respective compositions, clinical suitability, and long-term performance. Discussions encompass a range of factors including prosthetic space requirements, esthetic considerations, clinical challenges such as bruxism and temporomandibular joint issues, as well as patient-specific considerations such as age. Through comparative analyses, the chapter highlights the strengths and weaknesses of each material type, offering insights into their suitability for different clinical scenarios. The chapter concludes with a discussion on future trends and innovations, paving the way for continued advancements in full-arch restoration materials. Overall, this chapter aims to inform clinicians and researchers, facilitating informed decision making and enhancing patient outcomes in implant dentistry.

Keywords: full-arch, passive fit, hybrid materials, monolithic materials, implant restorations

1. Introduction

Full-arch implant restorations represent a pinnacle in modern dentistry, offering patients an unparalleled opportunity for functional rehabilitation and esthetic restoration [1]. As the demand for comprehensive solutions to edentulism continues to rise, the choice of materials in crafting these restorations becomes an essential element in achieving long-term success [2].

The landscape of dental materials has undergone a profound transformation over the years, with the emergence of both hybrid and monolithic options [3]. This chapter embarks on a journey through the dynamic debate surrounding the selection of materials for full-arch implant restorations, exploring the nuanced considerations that clinicians must navigate in the pursuit of optimal outcomes [4].

Historically, dental prosthetics were crafted from materials that prioritized durability and functionality [5]. However, the evolving expectations of patients, coupled with advancements in material science, have given rise to a spectrum of possibilities [6]. From the traditional layered composites to the modern monolithic zirconia, the array of choices can be both empowering and daunting [7].

As clinicians, we stand at a crossroads where decisions regarding material selection not only impact the mechanical properties of restorations but also influence the esthetic, biocompatible, and long-term performance aspects. This chapter aims to dissect the dichotomy between hybrid and monolithic materials, offering an in-depth analysis of their respective strengths, weaknesses, and the clinical scenarios where one may excel over the other.

Join us on this exploration of the materials that form the foundation of full-arch implant restorations, as we navigate the complexities, weigh the evidence, and consider the implications for the future of prosthetic dentistry.

2. Historical perspective

2.1 Early materials in full-arch restorations

The journey of full-arch restorations traces back to a time when dental prosthetics were primarily crafted from materials such as acrylic resins and metal alloys [8]. These early materials, though foundational, posed challenges in terms of esthetics, durability, and biocompatibility (**Figures 1** and **2**).

2.2 Rise of Porcelain-Fused-to-Metal (PFM) restorations

The advent of Porcelain-Fused-to-Metal (PFM) marked a significant shift in full-arch restorations, offering a balance between strength and esthetics [9]. The

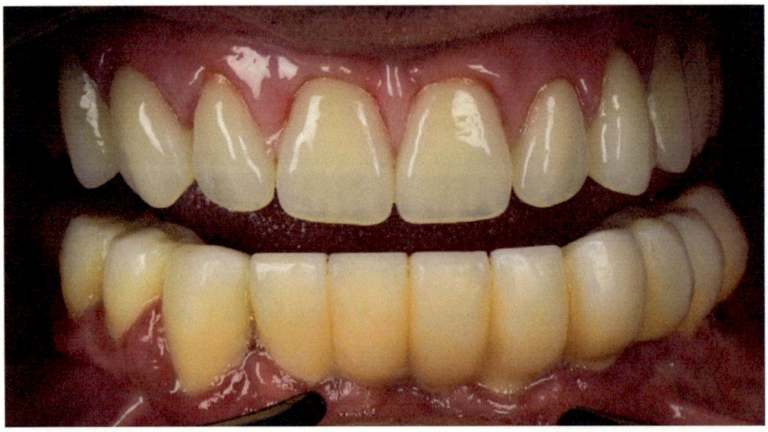

Figure 1.
Photo of a full-arch restoration with the first generation of layered composite on top of a cobalt-chrome frame.

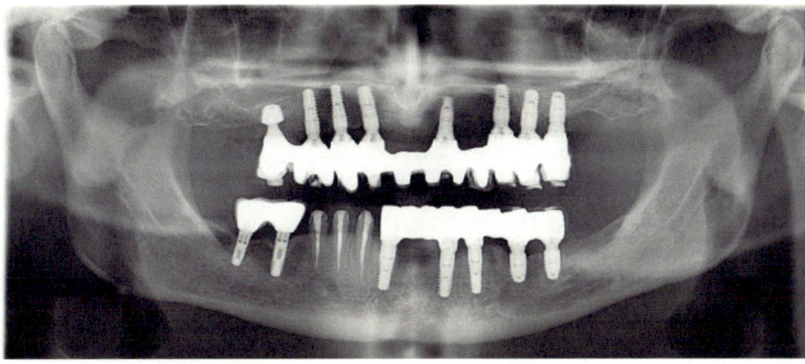

Figure 2.
*Orthopantomography of the same patient, as in **Figure 1**, for the final treatment assessment.*

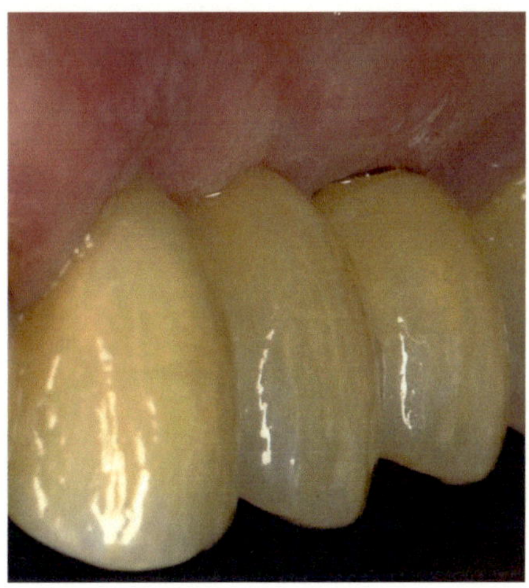

Figure 3.
Photos of a PFM restoration at the end of treatment.

metal substructure provided durability, while the porcelain overlay addressed esthetic concerns. PFM became a standard for many years, contributing to the restoration of edentulous arches (**Figure 3**).

2.3 Challenges and limitations of traditional materials

Despite their prevalence, traditional materials like PFM had inherent limitations. Issues such as chipping of porcelain, difficulties in achieving natural translucency, and the challenge of maintaining harmonious gingival contours prompted a quest for alternative solutions (**Figure 4**) [10].

2.4 Introduction of CAD/CAM technology

The introduction of Computer-Aided Design/Computer-Aided Manufacturing (CAD/CAM) technology revolutionized the field. This shift enabled the production of more precise (**Figure 5**) and patient-specific restorations, reducing the dependence on manual labor and facilitating the use of novel materials [11].

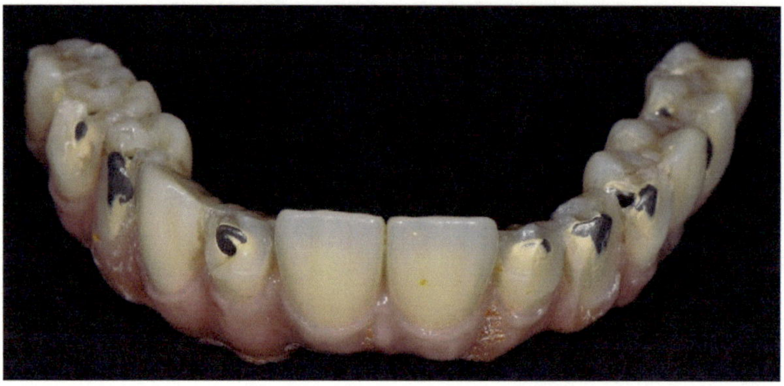

Figure 4.
PFM full-arch restoration with one of the most associated issues – The occurrence of porcelain chipping. There are several reasons (thickness of the porcelain layer, occlusal forces, brittleness of porcelain, incorrect occlusion or patient habits, misfit) why such problems may appear, and, in these cases, alternative materials must be chosen.

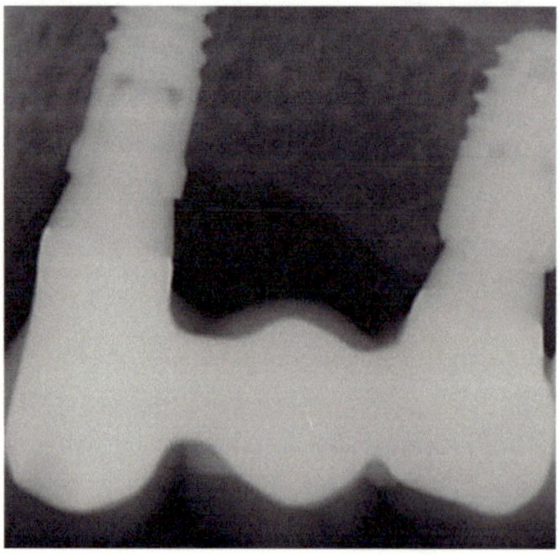

Figure 5.
Section of intraoral radiography of a restoration where can be seen the precision of the perfect fit of CAD/CAM restorations on implants.

2.5 Emergence of hybrid materials

Hybrid materials, combining a metal or zirconia framework with layered injected composites, entered the scene as a response to the limitations of traditional materials [12]. These materials aimed to capitalize on the strength of the substructure while enhancing esthetics through more lifelike surface layers (**Figure 6**).

2.6 Contemporary landscape and material diversity

In recent years, the landscape of full-arch restorations has become increasingly diverse. Materials like high-performance polymers, advanced ceramics, and monolithic multilayered zirconia (**Figure 7**) have gained popularity, offering clinicians a spectrum of options to address the unique needs of each case [13].

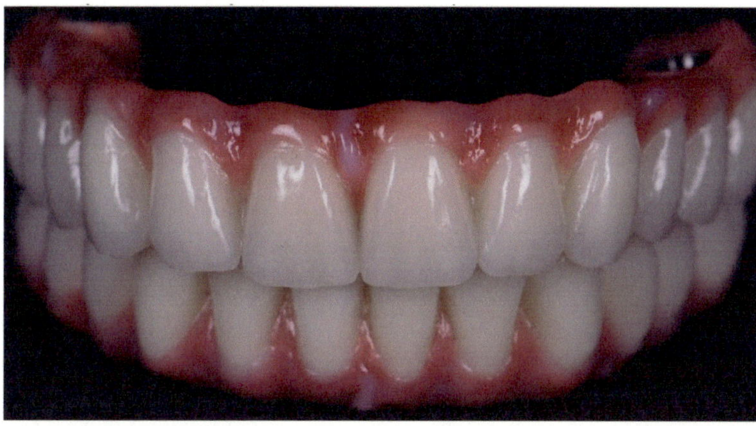

Figure 6.
Photo of a full-arch restoration with hybrid materials (latest injected composite on a milled metal frame) that emphasizes the improvement of the esthetic aspects of the restoration.

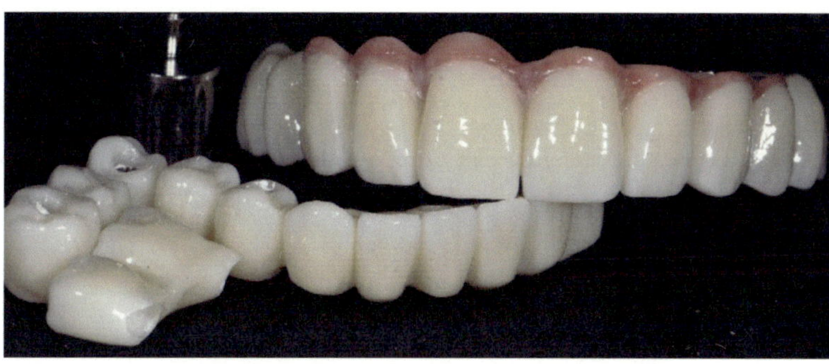

Figure 7.
Photo of several restorations made of the latest monolithic multilayered zirconia.

2.7 Impact on clinical outcomes

The evolution of materials in full-arch restorations has had a profound impact on clinical outcomes. Improved strength, enhanced esthetics, and a growing emphasis on patient-specific solutions have shaped the contemporary approach to full-arch implant restorations.

This historical perspective sets the stage for a comprehensive exploration of the contemporary debate between hybrid and monolithic materials, shedding light on the factors that have influenced their evolution and the implications for clinical practice.

3. Contemporary material options

3.1 Overview of material landscape

In the rapidly advancing field of full-arch implant restorations, clinicians find themselves at the intersection of innovation and tradition, tasked with navigating a diverse material landscape. The choice of materials is no longer a mere technical decision but a pivotal factor influencing the functional, esthetic, and long-term success of the restoration (**Table 1**).

3.2 Considerations in material selection

As clinicians navigate the landscape of hybrid and monolithic materials, several crucial considerations come into play. Patient preferences, the specific clinical context, and the overarching treatment goals should guide the decision-making process. This comprehensive overview sets the stage for a deeper exploration of the clinical considerations, esthetic implications, and long-term performance associated with the utilization of hybrid and monolithic materials in full-arch restorations.

Choosing the right materials for full-arch implant restorations is a critical decision for dentists. Essentially, we have two main options: hybrid materials and monolithic materials. Hybrid materials are like a blend of different layers, combining a strong base with detailed surface elements. On the other hand, monolithic materials are more straightforward, with a solid, uniform structure.

Materials	Hybrid materials	Monolithic materials
Definition	Hybrid materials represent a sophisticated amalgamation of strength and esthetics. This approach involves the strategic combination of a sturdy substructure, often composed of metals or high-strength ceramics like zirconia, with layered composite or ceramic materials for the visible surface.	Monolithic materials, in contrast, embody simplicity and strength. These materials, such as monolithic zirconia or other high-strength ceramics, maintain a uniform composition throughout the entire restoration.
Composition	The foundational strength of the hybrid lies in its substructure, which provides durability and support. This is then layered with composite materials or ceramics to achieve the desired esthetic appearance. The layering process allows for the customization of color, translucency, and surface texture, mimicking the natural dentition.	These restorations are typically milled or produced from a single block of material (**Figure 8**), ensuring homogeneity in strength and color. Monolithic zirconia, for instance, boasts exceptional durability and resistance to wear.
Advantages	*Esthetic versatility:* Layering techniques offer a broad spectrum of esthetic possibilities, enabling clinicians to achieve lifelike results. *Strength and support:* The robust substructure ensures the restoration's durability and stability. *Repairability:* In the event of minor issues, some hybrid restorations can be adjusted or repaired chairside.	*Strength and durability:* Monolithic materials offer high resistance to fractures and chipping due to their uniform composition. *Streamlined fabrication:* The manufacturing process is often quicker and more straightforward than the intricate layering involved in hybrids. *Consistency:* The entire restoration exhibits consistent color and strength.
Challenges	*Complex fabrication:* The intricate layering process demands skilled technicians and may lengthen the fabrication timeline. *Maintenance considerations:* The layered nature of hybrid materials may pose challenges in terms of wear and tear over time (**Figure 9**).	*Esthetic limitations:* While advancements have been made, monolithic materials may have limited variability in achieving natural esthetics compared to hybrids. *Adjustment challenges:* Chairside adjustments can be more challenging due to the hardness of the material.

Table 1.
Materials comparison: Hybrid vs. monolithic.

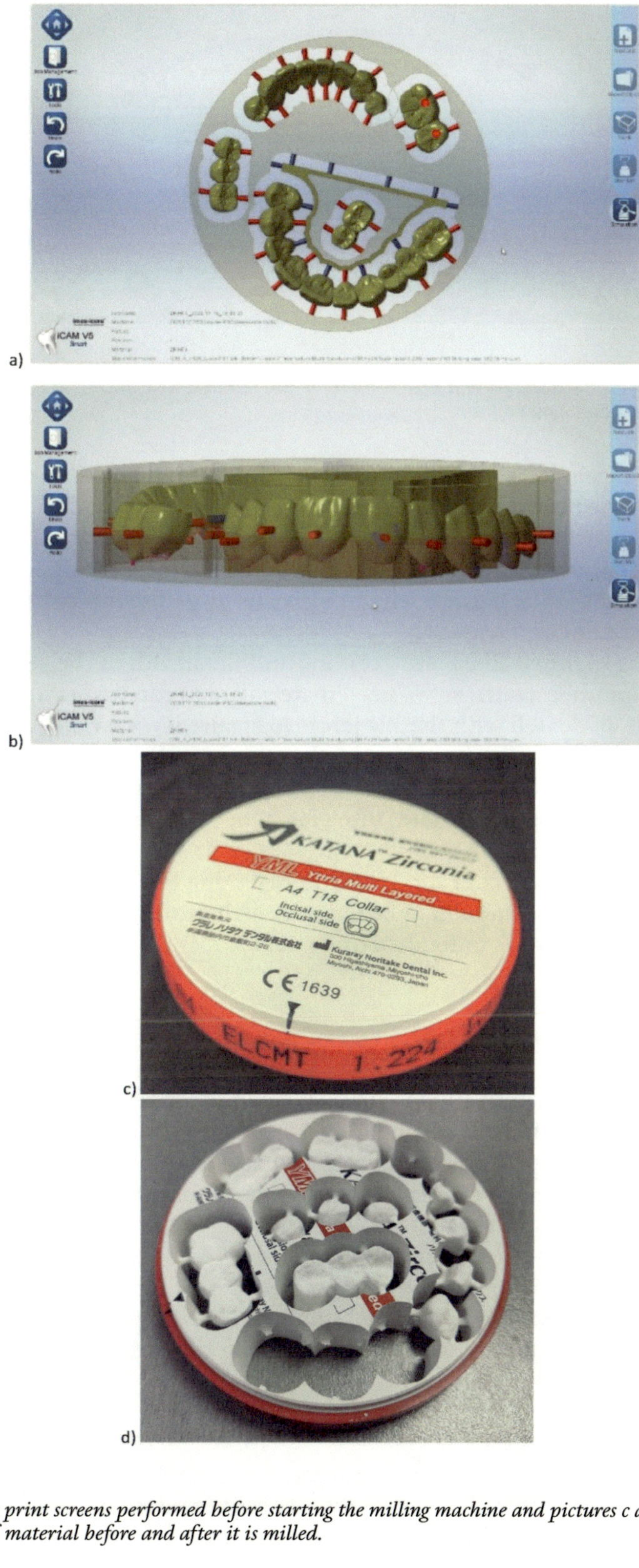

Figure 8.
Photos a and b are print screens performed before starting the milling machine and pictures c and d are examples of a single block of material before and after it is milled.

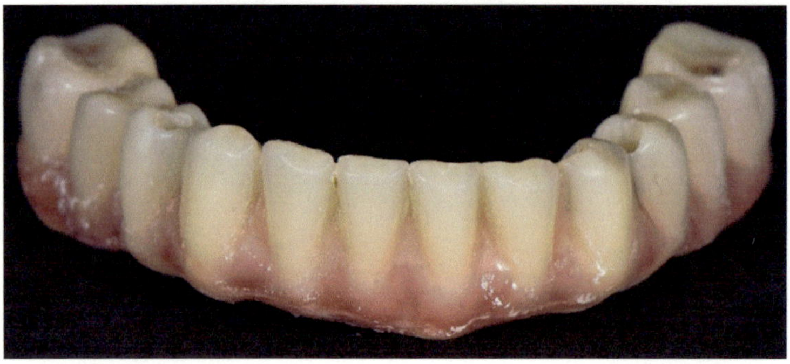

Figure 9.
Photo of a hybrid full-arch restoration that exposes the wear and tear over time because of the layered nature of hybrid materials composite on metal frame.

Now, why does this decision matter so much? Well, it is about tailoring the solution to each patient's unique needs. Think of it as fitting puzzle pieces together in the mouth.

First off, we consider the available space. Hybrid materials might require a bit more room due to their layered nature. Then, there's the esthetic aspect—ensuring the replacement teeth look natural. Hybrids give us more flexibility here, allowing for customization in color and texture.

We also factor in things like teeth grinding and the health of the jaw joints (TMJ). Some people grind their teeth, so we need materials that can withstand that. And the materials should work well with the jaw joints to ensure long-term health.

Considering the impact on opposing teeth—the ones the new implants will bite against—is crucial. We want a material that will not cause excessive wear and tear on these natural teeth. Patient age comes into play, too; younger and older mouths may require different considerations.

So, it is a bit like being a chef in a kitchen—selecting the right ingredients for the perfect dish. We want the implant to be durable, esthetically pleasing, and seamlessly integrated into each person's individual oral puzzle.

4. Clinical considerations

The choice between hybrid and monolithic materials is deeply influenced by several clinical factors. The patient's overall oral health, including the condition of existing teeth and supporting structures, is a pivotal consideration. The periodontal status, particularly the health of the gums and surrounding tissues, can influence the decision, with hybrid materials often offering advantages in achieving harmonious gingival contours. Restoration complexity, such as the number of missing teeth and the overall restoration design, plays a role in guiding the selection process. Additionally, understanding the patient's occlusal dynamics, including bite alignment and potential parafunctional habits, is critical in determining the most suitable material.

4.1 Prosthetic space

- *Definition and importance*: Prosthetic space refers to the available vertical and horizontal space within the oral cavity for accommodating dental restorations [14]. It encompasses the height and width required for fixed dental prostheses, considering factors such as adjacent teeth, occlusal clearance, and bone volume. The adequate availability of prosthetic space is crucial for determining the type of restoration that can be accommodated.

- *Influence on material selection*: Prosthetic space significantly influences the choice between hybrid and monolithic materials. Hybrid materials might necessitate more space due to their layered construction, whereas monolithic materials, being more conservative in space requirements, could be more suitable in cases with limited available space.

- *Diagnostic assessment*: Accurate measurement and assessment of prosthetic space involve thorough diagnostic procedures, including radiographic evaluation, digital impressions, and clinical measurements. These assessments aid in determining the feasibility of different restoration types and material choices based on the available space.

- *Treatment planning considerations*: Prosthetic space evaluation is a critical aspect of treatment planning for full-arch restorations. Clinicians must consider the ideal dimensions required for the chosen restoration type and material, ensuring a proper fit, functional occlusion, and long-term success.

- *Clinical challenges and solutions*: In cases of limited prosthetic space, clinicians may face challenges in selecting and designing appropriate restorations. Techniques such as minimal preparation or modification of the abutment teeth might be employed to optimize available space without compromising the restoration's integrity.

- *Long-term implications*: The consideration of prosthetic space extends to the long-term success of the restoration. Insufficient space can lead to complications such as poor fit, compromised occlusion, and potential mechanical failures. Adequate space ensures proper adaptation, stability, and functional harmony of the restoration within the oral environment (**Table 2**).

Aspect	Monolithic materials	Hybrid materials
Space requirements	Demand less space due to compact, single-block fabrication (See **Figure 10**)	Require more space for layered construction
Strength and durability	Exhibit exceptional strength and durability despite compactness	Offer good strength, may require meticulous handling
Fit and adaptation	Fit well within confined spaces without compromising integrity	May face challenges fitting in limited spaces
Esthetic customization	Limited esthetic customization but adequate natural appearance	Allow intricate customization for lifelike esthetics
Clinical considerations	Suitability for limited space cases, ensuring durable fit	Versatility in achieving detailed esthetics
Long-term implications	Proper adaptation within limited space ensures functional harmony	May face difficulties in cases with constrained space

Table 2.
Comparison of monolithic and hybrid materials in prosthetic space considerations.

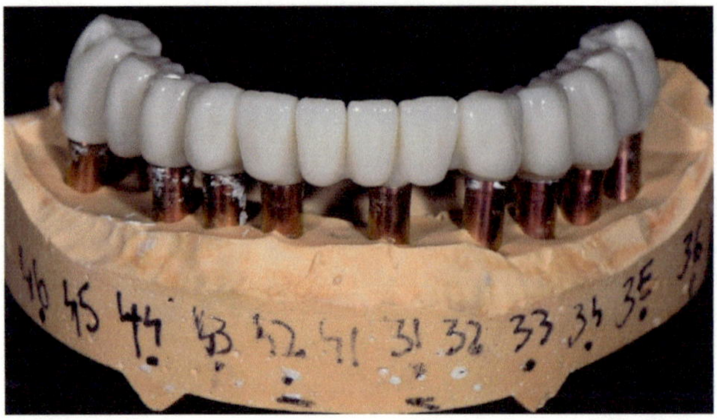

Figure 10.
Photo of a monolithic full-arch restoration where can be easily observed the suitability for limited space cases, ensuring long-term success.

4.2 Esthetic considerations

- *Importance of esthetics:* Esthetics serve as a cornerstone in full-arch restorations, influencing patient satisfaction, self-esteem, and overall treatment success. Achieving natural-looking teeth is paramount, especially in the anterior region, where visual prominence is heightened [15].

- *Material influence on esthetics:* The selection between monolithic and hybrid materials substantially influences the final esthetic outcome. Hybrid materials offer unparalleled versatility in replicating natural tooth characteristics [4]. This adaptability enables intricate color matching, translucency modulation, and surface texture emulation, ensuring a striking resemblance to natural dentition. Conversely, monolithic materials may exhibit limitations in precisely replicating the detailed esthetics of natural teeth due to their homogeneous structure [15].

- *Customization for natural appearance:* Hybrid materials stand out for their ability to achieve detailed customization, facilitating the recreation of the nuanced complexities of natural dentition [4]. Their diverse shades, translucency options, and surface textures allow for meticulous replication of natural teeth, ensuring seamless integration with adjacent dentition. However, monolithic materials, though lacking the intricate customization capabilities of hybrids, offer consistent and reliable uniformity, catering well to cases that demand durability over nuanced esthetics [16].

- *Patient expectations and satisfaction:* Understanding and aligning with patient expectations regarding esthetics are critical for successful full-arch restorations. Patients often harbor high expectations for a natural-looking smile [17]. Managing these expectations while considering the strengths and limitations of chosen materials is pivotal in achieving patient satisfaction and acceptance of the final esthetic outcome.

- *Longevity and stability of esthetic results:* Assessing the long-term stability and durability of esthetic outcomes is crucial [15]. Both monolithic and hybrid

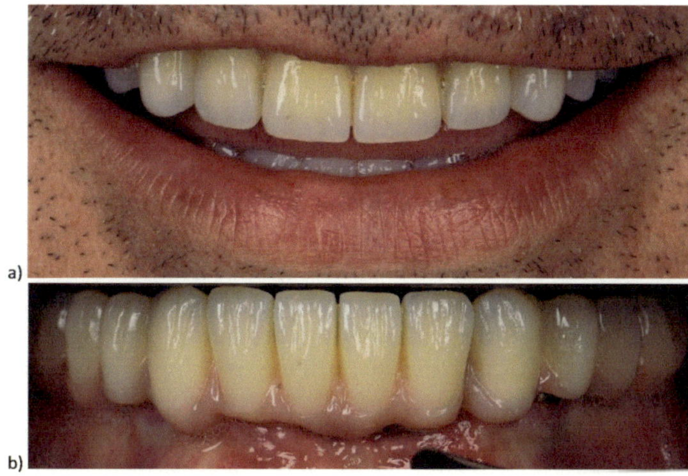

Figure 11.
Photos of a hybrid full-arch restoration that emphasizes the advantages of utilizing hybrid materials (the latest generation of injected composite) for achieving natural esthetics.

materials may provide satisfactory initial esthetic results, but considerations of long-term color stability, surface integrity, and wear resistance are paramount to ensure enduring esthetic appeal.

- *Clinical techniques and enhancements:* Beyond material choice, attention to clinical techniques significantly contributes to superior esthetic outcomes. Prudent tooth preparation, meticulous restoration design, precise shade matching, and attention to contouring and surface texture play pivotal roles in enhancing overall esthetics, irrespective of the chosen material type (**Figure 11**) [17].

5. Monolithic vs. hybrid materials in esthetic performance

5.1 Monolithic materials: esthetic integrity vs. uniformity

Proponents of monolithic materials advocate for their structural integrity and uniformity, attributing these characteristics to enhanced strength and resistance to fractures. The homogeneous composition of materials like zirconia or lithium disilicate offers consistent color and translucency throughout the restoration, ensuring durability and longevity. However, while these materials excel in strength, their limitations lie in the difficulty of achieving nuanced esthetic details. The uniform structure may impede the replication of natural tooth complexities, especially in mimicking fine color gradients and subtle surface textures. This uniformity can result in restorations that appear less natural in complex esthetic cases requiring intricate customization.

5.2 Hybrid materials: versatility for natural Esthetics

Advocates for hybrid materials emphasize their versatility in replicating natural tooth esthetics with precision. The layered construction, combining a strong substructure (e.g., zirconia or metal) with esthetic layers of ceramics or composite resins, offers unparalleled customization possibilities. This versatility allows for lifelike translucency, color variation, and intricate surface texture, closely resembling natural dentition. However, the layering technique, while enabling detailed customization, may introduce challenges such as potential chipping or delamination between layers, demanding meticulous fabrication and handling during adjustments.

The comparison between monolithic and hybrid materials for esthetic performance in full-arch restorations accentuates the trade-off between reliability and versatility. Monolithic materials, valued for their uniformity and durability, might compromise nuanced esthetic details, especially in complex cases. Hybrid materials, offering versatility for natural esthetics, may demand careful handling due to the layered construction but excel in replicating natural tooth complexities.

The decision hinges on balancing clinical requirements, patient expectations, and material capabilities. Monolithic materials, while providing strength and reliability, may be preferred for cases prioritizing durability over nuanced esthetics. Hybrid materials, though requiring meticulous handling, shine in cases where precise esthetic customization is crucial for achieving natural-looking outcomes.

5.3 Bruxism

- *Impact of bruxism:* Bruxism, characterized by teeth grinding or clenching, poses significant challenges in full-arch restorations [18]. The excessive occlusal forces exerted by bruxism can lead to increased mechanical stress on dental restorations, potentially compromising their longevity and structural integrity [19].

- *Material influence on bruxism:* In cases of bruxism, material selection plays a critical role in ensuring restoration durability. Monolithic materials, recognized for their high strength and resistance to fractures, are often preferred for bruxers [20]. These materials, like zirconia or high-strength ceramics, exhibit superior mechanical properties, providing better resistance against the abrasive forces associated with bruxism. Conversely, hybrid materials, despite their esthetic advantages, may be more susceptible to wear or damage due to their layered construction and varied material compositions.

- *Clinical management strategies:* Managing full-arch restorations in bruxism cases necessitates a comprehensive approach. Thorough occlusal analysis, precise occlusal adjustments, and occlusal splints play vital roles in mitigating the adverse effects of bruxism on restorations [19]. Additionally, meticulous polishing and surface treatments of restorations can enhance their wear resistance and reduce the likelihood of wear-induced complications.

- *Long-term implications:* Bruxism poses a considerable challenge in the long-term success of full-arch restorations [18]. The continuous occlusal forces exerted during bruxism may lead to wear, chipping, or fracture of restorative materials over time. Monitoring and regular follow-ups are crucial to detect and address potential complications early, ensuring the restoration's longevity in bruxism patients.

Bruxism significantly impacts full-arch restorations, necessitating careful consideration during material selection and clinical management. While monolithic materials offer superior strength and resistance to occlusal forces, they might be preferred for cases involving bruxism. However, comprehensive management strategies involving meticulous occlusal analysis and maintenance are vital for ensuring the long-term success of restorations in bruxism patients.

Monolithic materials, exemplified by zirconia, are distinguished by their exceptional strength and durability, making them highly resilient to fractures associated with bruxism [18, 19]. Their homogeneous structure contributes to enhanced material integrity, enabling greater resistance against wear and chipping caused by bruxing forces [19]. In clinical settings, monolithic materials often afford straightforward adaptability, requiring minimal adjustments and facilitating ease in managing occlusal discrepancies attributed to bruxism [20].

On the other hand, hybrid materials, characterized by their layered construction, present a nuanced scenario. While offering potential esthetic advantages, these materials might pose challenges in maintaining cohesive strength and durability under the continuous occlusal forces of bruxism. The layered composition in hybrid materials increases the susceptibility to delamination or fractures, potentially compromising their longevity and structural integrity, especially in cases of bruxism. Clinical adaptation with hybrid materials could demand meticulous handling and frequent adjustments, potentially posing challenges in managing the restoration's integrity under the continuous bruxing forces [19].

In summary, monolithic materials like zirconia demonstrate robust strength and durability, offering resilience against wear and fractures associated with bruxism. Their uniform structure and clinical adaptability might provide advantages in managing cases of bruxism. Conversely, hybrid materials, while potentially offering esthetic advantages, may pose challenges in maintaining material integrity and clinical adaptability in cases involving continuous bruxing forces.

5.4 TMJ issues

- *Impact of TMJ health:* The health of the temporomandibular joint (TMJ) holds significant importance in the success of full-arch restorations. TMJ disorders can affect occlusal stability, leading to challenges in treatment planning and execution [21].

- *Material influence on TMJ:* Material selection in full-arch restorations can significantly influence TMJ health. Monolithic materials, known for their uniformity and strength, might offer favorable occlusal stability and minimize adverse impacts on the TMJ [22]. Conversely, the layered construction of hybrid materials may require meticulous occlusal adjustments to ensure harmonious TMJ function, especially in cases with existing TMJ issues.

- *Occlusal considerations and treatment planning:* A thorough understanding of the patient's TMJ status is essential for comprehensive treatment planning in full-arch restorations. Accurate diagnostic methods, including imaging and occlusal analysis, aid in identifying TMJ-related issues and guide appropriate treatment strategies [23]. Occlusal adjustments and splint therapies might be necessary to manage TMJ-related symptoms and establish a stable occlusal relationship.

- *Clinical management strategies:* Careful consideration of occlusal factors and occlusal equilibration techniques can aid in minimizing TMJ-related complications in full-arch restorations [24]. Occlusal splints or other adjunctive therapies might be utilized to stabilize the occlusion and alleviate TMJ-related discomfort during the restoration process.

- *Long-term implications:* The impact of TMJ issues on full-arch restorations extends to their long-term success. Any occlusal discrepancies or untreated TMJ disorders may lead to discomfort, compromised function, and potential restoration failure over time. Regular follow-ups and monitoring of TMJ health are imperative for ensuring the stability and longevity of restorations.

The consideration of TMJ health is crucial in the planning and execution of full-arch restorations. Material selection, meticulous treatment planning, and clinical management strategies tailored to the patient's TMJ status are pivotal for minimizing TMJ-related complications and ensuring the long-term success of restorations (**Table 3**).

In summary, while monolithic materials like zirconia exhibit uniformity and strength, potentially contributing to improved occlusal stability and reduced impact on TMJ health, they might offer more straightforward clinical management in cases with existing TMJ issues. Conversely, hybrid materials, despite their esthetic advantages, may pose challenges in achieving optimal occlusal harmony and require meticulous adjustments, especially in patients with TMJ disorders.

5.5 Impact on opposing teeth

- *Influence of material type:* The choice of materials for full-arch restorations can significantly influence the impact on opposing dentition. Monolithic materials, known for their strength and hardness, have the potential to distribute occlusal forces evenly, minimizing wear on opposing natural teeth [25]. These materials, such as zirconia or high-strength ceramics, can maintain occlusal stability, reducing the likelihood of excessive wear or damage to opposing dentition.

- In contrast, hybrid materials, characterized by their layered construction, might present challenges in replicating the hardness and wear resistance

Factors	Monolithic materials	Hybrid materials
Strength and Uniformity	Monolithic materials, such as zirconia, offer uniformity and high strength, potentially contributing to improved occlusal stability and reduced impact on TMJ health.	Hybrid materials might require meticulous adjustments due to their layered construction, potentially posing challenges in achieving optimal occlusal harmony in cases with existing TMJ issues.
Occlusal Adaptation	The homogeneous structure of monolithic materials may aid in establishing stable occlusal relationships, potentially minimizing occlusal discrepancies related to TMJ disorders.	Layered construction in hybrid materials could necessitate extensive occlusal adjustments to achieve harmonious occlusion, especially in cases with TMJ issues, potentially posing challenges in achieving stable occlusal relationships.
Clinical Management	Monolithic materials might offer ease in occlusal adjustments and clinical adaptability, potentially aiding in managing occlusal discrepancies associated with TMJ disorders.	Clinical management with hybrid materials may require meticulous handling and comprehensive occlusal analysis to establish stable occlusal relationships in patients with TMJ issues.

Table 3.
Comparison: monolithic vs. hybrid materials in relation to TMJ issues.

comparable to natural teeth or monolithic restorations [25]. The variations in material properties between layers in hybrid restorations may potentially result in increased wear on opposing teeth due to differential hardness or surface characteristics.

- *Clinical observations and considerations:* Clinical observations suggest that monolithic restorations exhibit favorable wear properties, providing minimal abrasiveness to opposing dentition [26]. The hardness and structural integrity of monolithic materials contribute to reduced wear rates on natural teeth when compared to hybrid restorations.

- However, hybrid materials, particularly those with softer veneering layers or varying compositions, might exhibit increased wear characteristics, potentially causing accelerated wear on opposing natural teeth [26]. The differential wear properties between hybrid layers and natural dentition could lead to uneven wear patterns and potentially compromise the longevity of the restoration.

- *Long-term implications:* Considering the long-term implications, monolithic materials tend to offer a more favorable impact on opposing dentition, exhibiting minimal wear on natural teeth, and maintaining occlusal harmony. On the contrary, the potential for increased wear with hybrid materials might require careful monitoring and regular assessment to manage any accelerated wear issues on opposing dentition [27].

The choice between monolithic and hybrid materials for full-arch restorations holds significance in their impact on opposing dentition. Monolithic materials, with their superior hardness and wear characteristics, tend to have a more favorable impact, minimizing wear on natural teeth. Conversely, hybrid materials, due to their variable composition and potential differences in hardness, might present challenges, potentially leading to accelerated wear on opposing dentition.

Monolithic materials, with their inherent hardness and durability like natural teeth, tend to have a more favorable impact on opposing dentition, exhibiting minimal wear over time. Conversely, hybrid materials, with potential differences in hardness between layers, may present challenges in mimicking the wear characteristics of natural teeth, potentially causing accelerated wear on opposing dentition.

The debate between monolithic and hybrid materials concerning the impact on opposing teeth in full-arch restorations highlights the superiority of monolithic materials in minimizing wear on natural dentition. Their inherent hardness and wear resistance qualities offer sustained occlusal harmony, contrasting with potential challenges presented by hybrid materials, especially in replicating natural dentition hardness and wear characteristics.

5.6 Patient age considerations

- *Definition and importance:* Patient age plays a pivotal role in the selection of materials for full-arch restorations. Monolithic materials, like zirconia or high-strength ceramics, are characterized by exceptional hardness and wear resistance, qualities advantageous for older patients prone to increased occlusal wear or age-related changes. Hybrid materials, while offering esthetic flexibility, may present challenges in replicating natural dentition hardness uniformly across layers, potentially affecting long-term performance in older individuals.

- *Influence on material selection:* Monolithic materials, due to their robustness and durability, emerge as favorable options for older patients or those experiencing age-related occlusal changes. The inherent hardness and wear resistance of monolithic materials offers enhanced longevity and reduced wear on restorations, accommodating increased occlusal forces associated with aging. In contrast, the variable properties between layers in hybrid restorations might pose challenges in mimicking natural dentition hardness in older patients, potentially impacting long-term performance [28].

- *Diagnostic assessment:* Accurate evaluation of patient age and associated factors is essential in material selection for full-arch restorations. Monolithic materials demonstrate advantages in sustaining durability and resisting wear in older patients with potentially compromised dentition due to age-related factors. Conversely, hybrid materials might necessitate comprehensive diagnostic assessments to gauge their suitability in managing age-related occlusal changes and potential wear discrepancies [28].

- *Clinical implications:* Monolithic materials provide reliable solutions for older patients, ensuring longevity and reduced wear on restorations, aligning well with age-related occlusal demand. However, hybrid materials might require meticulous clinical management and closer monitoring, especially concerning potential wear discrepancies and challenges in replicating natural dentition hardness, particularly in older individuals [28].

In evaluating patient age considerations for full-arch restorations, monolithic materials demonstrate superior durability and wear resistance, making them more suitable for older individuals with increased occlusal demands and age-related changes. On the contrary, while offering esthetic advantages, the variable composition of hybrid materials might pose challenges in managing age-related occlusal changes and wear discrepancies in older patients.

Considering patient age as a crucial factor, the selection of monolithic materials for full-arch restorations emerges as a preferred option for older individuals. The robustness and durability of monolithic materials offer enhanced longevity and reduced wear, addressing the challenges associated with age-related occlusal changes, compared to potential concerns posed by hybrid materials.

6. Strengths and weaknesses of hybrid and monolithic materials

6.1 Hybrid materials

- *Strengths:* Hybrid materials excel in esthetic versatility, allowing for detailed customization to achieve natural-looking results. They also offer repairability, enabling chairside adjustments for minor issues.

- *Weaknesses:* The fabrication process can be complex, demanding skilled technicians and potentially extending the timeline. Maintenance challenges may arise due to the layered nature of these materials.

DOI: http://dx.doi.org/10.5772/intechopen.114307

6.2 Monolithic materials

- *Strengths:* Monolithic materials boast high durability throughout, offering resistance to fractures and chipping. The simplified fabrication process is quicker and more straightforward than that of hybrid materials.

- *Weaknesses:* Esthetic limitations may pose challenges in achieving intricate appearance details. Chairside adjustments can be more complex due to the material's hardness.

7. Biocompatibility and tissue response

Biocompatibility and tissue response to different materials form a critical aspect of full-arch implant restorations. Hybrid materials, with their combination of substructure and layered components, interact dynamically with the oral environment. Monolithic materials, being uniform throughout, offer a different interaction profile. Understanding the biocompatibility of each material ensures long-term integration and minimizes the risk of adverse reactions within the oral cavity.

In the context of hybrid and monolithic restorations, considerations of biocompatibility extend beyond material composition to encompass how each restoration type interacts with surrounding tissues. The response of the gingiva, potential inflammatory reactions, and overall tissue health are crucial factors in the decision-making process. Clinicians must weigh these aspects carefully to ensure the selected material promotes not only functional success but also a healthy and harmonious relationship with the oral environment.

8. Case studies

Hybrid materials, characterized by layered structures as can be observed in **Table 4**, present a dynamic interplay between opacity changes and hygiene considerations. Over time, these materials may undergo opacity alterations due to factors like wear, staining, or modifications in composition. This increased porosity creates microscopic spaces, raising concerns about bacterial accumulation. In contrast, monolithic materials, exemplified also in **Table 4**, embody stability and resilience in the face of hygiene variations. Their opacity remains consistently stable over time, providing a reliable esthetic profile.

The consideration of Vertical Occlusion Dimension (DVO) is pivotal in the success of full-arch restorations. DVO encompasses the dynamic interplay of occlusal forces during various functional movements, including chewing and speech. The choice of materials must align with the dynamic nature of occlusion, ensuring that the restoration can withstand and distribute forces harmoniously. This consideration is particularly crucial for full-arch restorations, where occlusal demands are distributed across multiple teeth. The selection of materials for full-arch restorations involves a careful balance of various factors.

Each material option, whether traditional such as porcelain-fused-to-metal (PFM) or contemporary like zirconia or lithium disilicate, comes with its unique set of characteristics. Evaluating the patient's specific needs, occlusal scheme, and esthetic preferences becomes imperative. Recent advancements in materials, such as

Case	Material type	Pros	Cons
Prosthetic space	Hybrid	• Offers layering for esthetic customization • Potential for easier repairs and adjustments	• Requires more space due to layered construction • Susceptible to delamination or chipping
	Monolithic	• Conservative in-space requirements • Superior durability and resistance to fractures	• Limited esthetic versatility • Challenging repairs or adjustments
Esthetics	Hybrid	• Enhanced esthetic adaptability and lifelike translucency • Natural appearance like natural dentition	• Potential for color discrepancies between layers • Proneness to wear variations over time
	Monolithic	• Uniform color and translucency resembling natural teeth • Robustness and resistance to wear	• Limited customization in esthetics • Challenges in achieving lifelike translucency
Bruxism	Hybrid	• Potential for absorbing forces due to layered composition • Esthetic layer provides chipping resistance	• Susceptible to wear discrepancies between layers • Possible delamination in high-stress situations
	Monolithic	• High resistance to fractures and wear • Superior durability under occlusal forces	• Limited ability to absorb forces like hybrid materials • Challenging repairs in case of damage
TMJ Issues	Hybrid	• Layered construction offers potential shock absorption • Esthetic layers enhance restoration appearance	• Possibility of wear differences between layers • Risk of chipping or delamination
	Monolithic	• Superior strength and resilience against occlusal forces • Reduced risk of wear discrepancies	• Limited shock-absorbing capability compared to hybrids • Potential challenges in achieving optimal esthetics
Impact on Opposing Teeth	Hybrid	• Esthetic layer potentially minimizes wear on opposing teeth • Potential for shock absorption	• Varying wear characteristics between layers • Risk of chipping or delamination
	Monolithic	• Consistent wear properties resembling natural dentition • Reduced wear on opposing teeth	• Limited shock absorption compared to hybrid materials • Challenges in esthetics customization
Patient Age Considerations	Hybrid	• Esthetic customization for age-related changes • Layered construction offers potential wear adaptation	• Variable wear characteristics between layers • Susceptibility to wear discrepancies in aged dentition
	Monolithic	• Superior durability and wear resistance in aged dentition • Consistent wear properties	• Limited customization for age-related changes • Potential challenges in managing wear discrepancies

Table 4.
Comparison: monolithic vs. hybrid materials – conclusions.

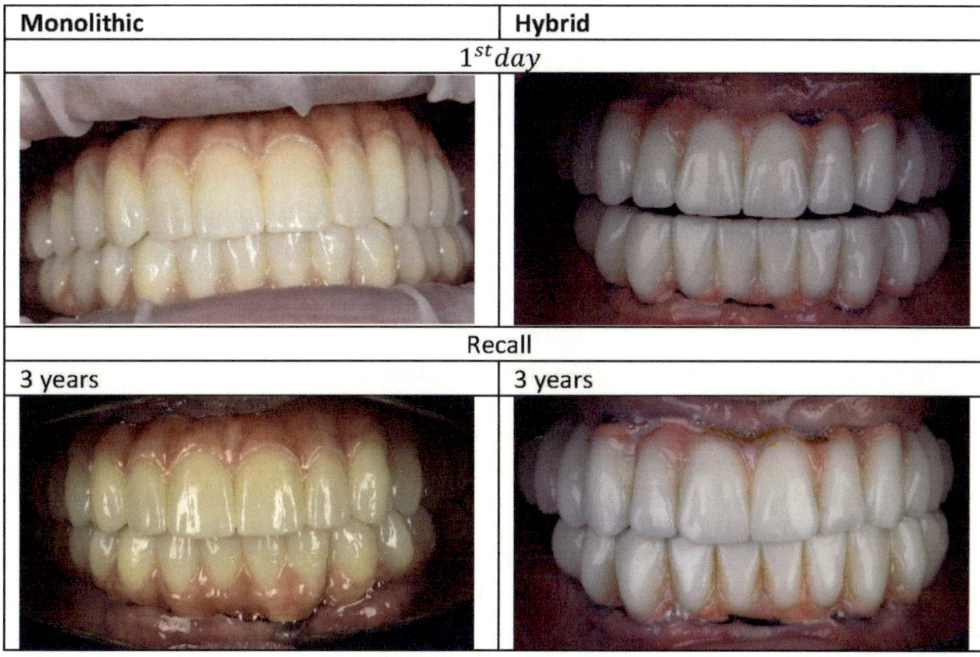

Figure 12.
Two case studies with full-arch restorations on both maxillary and mandible, from the first meeting until the last recall.

high-performance polymers and bioactive composites, offer promising alternatives, introducing a new dimension to material selection (**Figure 12**).

A trade-off analysis between materials is inherent in the decision-making process. Traditional materials may provide durability but could pose challenges in achieving optimal esthetics. On the other hand, newer materials with enhanced esthetics might require careful consideration of their mechanical properties and long-term performance. Finding the delicate balance between esthetics, resistance to wear, and overall longevity is a central theme in the trade-off discussions, necessitating a personalized approach for each patient. The discussion underscores the importance of individualized treatment planning for full-arch restorations. Tailoring the material selection to each patient's unique requirements, considering their occlusal dynamics, esthetic expectations, and potential lifestyle factors, is paramount. This approach ensures that the chosen materials not only meet immediate needs but also contribute to the long-term success and satisfaction of the restoration.

The choice of Zirconia restorations glued to a titanium milled bar represents a contemporary approach, combining the strength of Zirconia with the lightweight and biocompatibility of titanium. This material pairing aims to offer a harmonious blend of durability, resistance to corrosion, and biocompatibility. The selection hinges on achieving a balance between the mechanical properties of Zirconia and the favorable characteristics of titanium. This technique facilitates resistant restoration for patients with DVO bigger than 14 mm. A monolithic restoration would be too heavy, and a hybrid restoration such as PFMs is not reliable on such medical cases because there it is a lack of resistance.

9. Future trends and innovations

9.1 Emerging materials and technologies

The ever-evolving landscape of dental materials and technologies continues to drive innovation in full-arch restorations. Emerging materials, such as high-performance polymers, nano-ceramics, and bioactive composites, are gaining traction, aiming to combine strength, esthetics, and biocompatibility. These materials showcase improved mechanical properties and enhanced esthetic possibilities, offering promising alternatives in the quest for optimal restorative solutions.

9.2 Digital advancements and CAD/CAM integration

The advent of digital dentistry has revolutionized the fabrication process for full-arch restorations. Advanced CAD/CAM technologies streamline workflow, enabling precise digital impressions, design, and manufacturing of restorations. Integration with intraoral scanners, 3D printing, and virtual treatment planning optimizes accuracy, efficiency, and patient satisfaction. Future advancements are anticipated to further refine these technologies, enhancing precision and expanding material options.

9.2.1 Biomimetic and bioactive approaches

Innovations inspired by biomimicry and bioactivity are shaping the future of restorative materials [29, 30]. Biomimetic designs aim to replicate natural tooth structure and function, fostering enhanced integration and functionality within the oral environment. Bioactive materials, capable of stimulating tissue regeneration or remineralization, hold promise in fostering improved interactions at the restoration-to-tooth interface, potentially enhancing longevity and biocompatibility.

9.2.2 Personalized and regenerative dentistry

The shift toward personalized dentistry encompasses tailored treatment approaches based on individual patient characteristics [31]. Regenerative therapies, including tissue engineering and biologically driven approaches, are being explored to restore lost or damaged tissues around dental implants. This personalized approach aims to optimize treatment outcomes, promoting natural tissue regeneration and improving long-term success rates.

9.2.3 Implications for clinical practice

The integration of these evolving trends and innovations into clinical practice holds immense potential. Clinicians embracing these advancements are poised to offer enhanced treatment options, improved patient experiences, and long-lasting restorations. Continual education and adaptation to emerging technologies will be instrumental in leveraging these innovations to their full potential, ultimately benefiting both clinicians and patients.

10. Conclusion

The journey through the realm of full-arch restorations unveils a nuanced debate surrounding the selection of materials, notably between monolithic and hybrid compositions. These deliberations encompass a spectrum of clinical, functional, and esthetic considerations, shaping the paradigm of modern restorative dentistry.

Material landscape evolution: The historical trajectory illustrates a progression in materials from conventional options to contemporary choices. This evolution has pivoted toward the dichotomy of monolithic and hybrid materials, each offering distinct advantages and challenges in the landscape of full-arch restorations.

Clinical considerations and material selection: Clinical decision making is pivotal, influenced by multifaceted factors such as prosthetic space, occlusal dynamics, bruxism, TMJ status, opposing dentition, and patient age. Monolithic materials, epitomized by their robustness and wear resistance, are favored in scenarios necessitating durability and reduced wear on restorations, notably in older patients or those with higher occlusal demands. Hybrid materials, while presenting esthetic adaptability, may require meticulous management and closer scrutiny, especially concerning replicating natural dentition characteristics and managing occlusal challenges.

Strengths and weaknesses: Monolithic materials shine in their exceptional hardness, durability, and ability to mirror natural dentition wear characteristics, ensuring long-term stability and reduced wear on opposing teeth. Conversely, hybrid materials offer versatility in esthetics but might introduce challenges in uniform wear properties and longevity due to the variable composition across layers.

Esthetics, biocompatibility, and future implications: Esthetic considerations, biocompatibility, and ongoing technological advancements play pivotal roles in shaping the trajectory of material choices. Hybrid materials, with their esthetic potential, offer customizable options, while advancements aim to bridge the gap between strength and esthetics.

Patient-centric approach: The chapter underscores the paramount importance of an individualized patient-centric approach in material selection. Tailoring choices based on patient-specific factors ensures optimal outcomes, emphasizing the necessity of precise diagnosis, treatment planning, and meticulous execution.

In essence, while the debate between monolithic and hybrid materials persists, the selection must align with the specific clinical scenario and patient needs. Monolithic materials dominate in offering durability and reduced wear, especially in aged or occlusal-demanding patients, while hybrid materials present esthetic versatility but demand careful clinical handling. The future promises continued innovation, aiming to amalgamate strength, esthetics, and clinical adaptability, shaping the trajectory of full-arch restorations in restorative dentistry.

Author details

Ioan Achim Borsanu[1,2], Ralph-Alexandru Erdelyi[2,3], Laura Rusu[1], Sergiu Manuel Antonie[1,2] and Emanuel Adrian Bratu[1,2]*

1 "Victor Babes" University of Medicine and Pharmacy, Timisoara, Romania

2 Prof. Dr. Bratu Dental Clinic Dental Experts, Timisoara, Romania

3 Polytechnic University of Timisoara, Romania

*Address all correspondence to: ebratu@umft.ro

References

[1] Shillingburg HT, Sather DA, Cain JR, Mitchell DL, Blanco LJ, Kessler JC. Fundamentals of Fixed Prosthodontics. USA: Quintessence Publishing; 2012

[2] Abou-Ayash S, Strasding M, Rücker G, Att W. Impact of prosthetic material on mid-and long-term outcome of dental implants supporting single crowns and fixed partial dentures: A systematic review and meta-analysis. European Journal of Oral Implantology. 2017;**10**(Suppl. 1):47-65

[3] Furtado de Mendonca A, Shahmoradi M, Gouvêa CVDD, De Souza GM, Ellakwa A. Microstructural and mechanical characterization of CAD/CAM materials for monolithic dental restorations. Journal of Prosthodontics. 2019;**28**(2):e587-e594

[4] Al-Haj Husain N, Özcan M, Molinero-Mourelle P, Joda T. Clinical performance of partial and full-coverage fixed dental restorations fabricated from hybrid polymer and ceramic CAD/CAM materials: A systematic review and meta-analysis. Journal of Clinical Medicine. 2020;**9**(7):2107. Available from: https://www.mdpi.com/journal/jcm

[5] Bayne SC, Ferracane JL, Marshall GW, Marshall SJ, Van Noort R. The evolution of dental materials over the past century: Silver and gold to tooth color and beyond. Journal of Dental Research. 2019;**98**(3):257-265

[6] Ahmad I. Compobond: Evolution of a new restorative dental material. Cosmetic Dent Eng. 2011;**2**:26-37

[7] Schmalz G, Arenholt-Bindslev D. Biocompatibility of Dental Materials. Vol. 1. Berlin: Springer; 2009

[8] Delucchi F, De Giovanni E, Pesce P, Bagnasco F, Pera F, Baldi D, et al. Framework materials for full-arch implant-supported rehabilitations: A systematic review of clinical studies. Materials. 2021;**14**(12):3251

[9] Walter M, Reppel PD, Böning K, Freesmeyer WB. Six-year follow-up of titanium and high-gold porcelain-fused-to-metal fixed partial dentures. Journal of Oral Rehabilitation. 1999;**26**(2):91-96

[10] Saeed F, Muhammad N, Khan AS, Sharif F, Rahim A, Ahmad P, et al. Prosthodontics dental materials: From conventional to unconventional. Materials Science and Engineering: C. 2020;**106**:110167

[11] Rexhepi I, Santilli M, D'Addazio G, Tafuri G, Manciocchi E, Caputi S, et al. Clinical applications and mechanical properties of CAD-CAM materials in restorative and prosthetic dentistry: A systematic review. Journal of Functional Biomaterials. 2023;**14**(8):431

[12] Duarte S, Sartori N, Phark JH. Ceramic-reinforced polymers: CAD/CAM hybrid restorative materials. Current Oral Health Reports. 2016;**3**:198-202

[13] Powers JM, Wataha JC. Dental Materials-E-Book: Foundations and Applications. USA: Elsevier Health Sciences; 2015

[14] Carpentieri J, Greenstein G, Cavallaro J. Hierarchy of restorative space required for different types of dental implant prostheses. The Journal of the American Dental Association. 2019;**150**(8):695-706

[15] Aschheim KW. Esthetic Dentistry: A Clinical Approach to Techniques and Materials. USA: Elsevier Health Sciences; 2014

[16] Sha RK. The Concepts of Color Matching and Shade Selection in Prosthodontics. Lucknow: Book Rivers; 2021

[17] Ahmad I. Protocols for Predictable Aesthetic Dental Restorations. UK: John Wiley & Sons; 2008

[18] Manfredini D, Poggio CE. Prosthodontic planning in patients with temporomandibular disorders and/or bruxism: A systematic review. The Journal of Prosthetic Dentistry. 2017;**117**(5):606-613

[19] Manfredini D, Ahlberg J, Lobbezoo F. Bruxism definition: Past, present, and future–what should a prosthodontist know? The Journal of Prosthetic Dentistry. 2022;**128**(5):905-912

[20] Miotto CS, Vieira GF, Firsoff EFO, Puliti E, Marques AP, Greven M. Comparative effects of dental treatment and two different physical therapy interventions in individuals with bruxism: A randomized clinical trial. Journal of Clinical Medical Research. 2021;**3**(6):1-15

[21] Al-Ani Z, Gray RJ. Temporomandibular Disorders: A Problem-Based Approach. UK: John Wiley & Sons; 2021

[22] Hazra R, Srivastava A, Kumar D, Khattak A. Current trends in temporomandibular disorder management: A prosthodontist's perspective. Journal of Dentistry Defense Section. 2022;**16**(2):146-150

[23] Minervini G, Fiorillo L, Russo D, Lanza A, D'Amico C, Cervino G, et al. Prosthodontic treatment in patients with temporomandibular disorders and orofacial pain and/or bruxism: A review of the literature. Prosthesis. 2022;**4**(2):253-262

[24] Türp JC, Strub JR. Prosthetic rehabilitation in patients with temporomandibular disorders. The Journal of Prosthetic Dentistry. 1996;**76**(4):418-423

[25] Bhandari S. Outcome of single maxillary complete dentures opposing mandibular teeth: A need to introspect on the prosthodontic treatment protocol. The Journal of the Indian Prosthodontic Society. 2016;**16**(1):15

[26] Khan MS, Raza M, Khan H, Zubair N, Rahman EU, Afridi S. Assessment of supraeruption of teeth affecting prosthodontics rehabilitation in different segments of opposing arch: Assessment of supraeruption of teeth. Pakistan Journal of Health Sciences. 2022;**3**(4):96-100

[27] Klineberg I, Eckert S. Functional Occlusion in Restorative Dentistry and Prosthodontics. Olanda: Elsevier Health Sciences; 2015

[28] Buser R, Yue Q, Zimmermann P, Suter V, Abou-Ayash S, Schimmel M. Prosthodontic solutions for elderly patients. Forum Implantologicum. 2018;**14**:130-140. DOI: 10.3290/iti.fi.45661

[29] Magne P, Douglas WH. Rationalization of esthetic restorative dentistry based on biomimetics. Journal of Esthetic and Restorative Dentistry. 1999;**11**(1):5-15

[30] Goudouri OM, Kontonasaki E, Theocharidou A, Papadopoulou L, Chatzistavrou X, Koidis P, et al. In vitro bioactivity studies of sol-gel derived dental ceramics/bioactive glass composites in periodically renewed biomimetic solution. Bioceramics Development and Applications. 2011;**1**:1-4

[31] Amrollahi P, Shah B, Seifi A, Tayebi L. Recent advancements in regenerative dentistry: A review. Materials Science and Engineering: C. 2016;**69**:1383-1390

Chapter 8

Composite Dental Implants: A Future Restorative Approach

Alexandra Roi, Ciprian Roi, Codruța Victoria Țigmeanu and Mircea Riviș

Abstract

The introduction of composites and dental materials in the implantology field has shown an important increase in the past years. The restorative approaches using dental implants are currently a desirable option for edentulous patients. Since their introduction in dentistry, dental implants have proven to be a reliable option for restabling the functions and esthetics of certain areas. Characteristics such as high biocompatibility, nontoxicity, and high corrosion resistance have been key factors for their worldwide acceptance. In time, researchers aimed to improve their qualities by manufacturing the implants using various materials that could improve the interaction between the bone and implant. Although, until now, dental implant materials were limited to the use of single or coated metals, there are certain limitations that current studies aimed to overcome by introducing a new category, the composite dental implants. With this new category, the mechanical characteristics can be designed in order for their integration and further functions to have a positive outcome. This chapter describes the use of composite dental implants as a restorative prosthetic option, their advantages, and physicochemical and osteointegration properties as future approaches for restorative prosthetic rehabilitation.

Keywords: composite dental implants, prosthetic restorations, osteointegration, biocompatibility, restorative dentistry

1. Introduction

Dental implants have increased in popularity and are nowadays among the first options for prosthetic restoration of partially edentulous or total edentulous patients. They have been used as artificial tooth roots that can support prosthetic restorations, starting from fixed single crowns and ending with removable dentures.

Their clinical use has been for over 30 years [1], providing important progress for dental and maxillofacial surgery as further prosthetic treatment approaches, as their use can improve the local restoration or represent a support for several orthodontic appliances.

From the research results provided by Brånemark and others [2–7] regarding the process of osteointegration of dental implants, the election material so far was titanium and titanium alloys due to their high biocompatibility, osteointegration induction, high resistance to corrosion, and other excellent mechanical properties. Hence, these are implied for correct substitution of the dental root. Until recently, this type of material was considered the gold standard for the manufacture of dental implants, having the main target to achieve a direct connection between the bone and the implant in order to ensure long-term resistance, fulfilling the future functions of a prosthesis [8]. The results of using titanium dental implants have been quantified, and the success rate is high, reporting no differences between the followed clinical protocol [9]. However, the implant failure cases that implied the removal of the dental implant were mainly the consequence of peri-implantitis, caused by the colonization of anaerobic micro-organisms on the implant surfaces [10].

As currently patients require fast treatment that includes quick implant placement and healing, followed by an immediate load for a functional prosthetic outcome, for the titanium implant in order to fulfill these requirements, their osteointegration and the entire dynamic process require at least 3 to 6 months for local healing and inducing the cellular process for osteointegration [11]. Also, reports show that, in the case of titanium implants, the diffusion of the metallic ions, as a consequence of the exposure of the metal surface to electrolytes, can induce an immune reaction (a type IV reaction), targeting the implant [12–14]. A problem can be represented by the elasticity modulus, being higher compared to the alveolar bone, **a** fact that can result in the failure of the implant as a consequence of inefficient stress shielding [15].

The research focusing on the development of materials, especially biomaterials and composites, has provided important information related to their use and applicability in dentistry and implantology. By introducing these classes of biomaterials such as ceramics, glass ceramics, hydroxyapatite, or polyetheretherketone (PEEK), their advantages for clinical applications have quickly transformed them into an alternative to the use of titanium implants. Improving the quality of the dental implants and influencing the future of implant-prosthetic restorations, this chapter aims to provide valuable information related to the use of composite implants as a treatment option.

2. Dental implants—biomechanical properties and osteointegration

2.1 Biomechanical properties of dental implants

A dental implant is considered a medical device with the main role of replacing a missing tooth. As a consequence, the physical, chemical, and biological characteristics of an implant should be correctly adjusted in order to stimulate and sustain the osteointegration process, as well as the future forces that will be directly absorbed and distributed in the area of the bone-implant interface [16]. While aiming to restore an edentation with the help of an implant prosthetic restoration, the clinician must take into consideration the biomechanical aspects of the two components of an implant: the screw and the abutment (**Figure 1**). Being a foreign dispositive that will be in contact with the human bone (the screw) and the oral soft tissue (the abutment), it is a desiderate to be integrated and accepted in order to be functional [17].

The main goal in implantology is to achieve the osteointegration process of the placed implant, in order to become stable and retained in the alveolar bone, to form a new bone-implant interface for further functional forces to be properly distributed.

The bone is an important tissue structure that is responsible for movement, protection, and support in the entire body. It has an organic component represented by collagen (types I, III, and IV) and fibrillin and an inorganic component represented

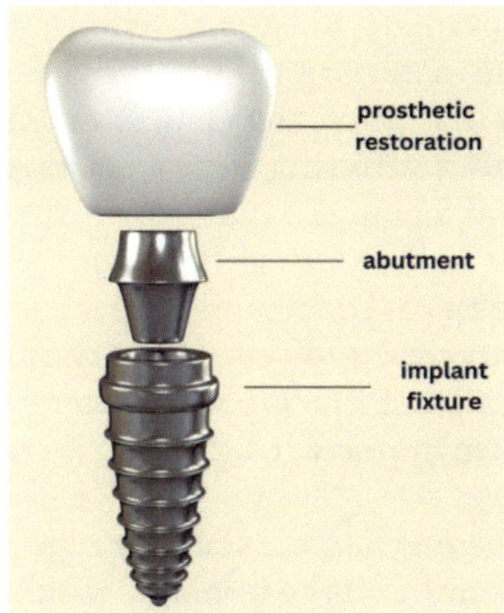

Figure 1.
Basic implant components.

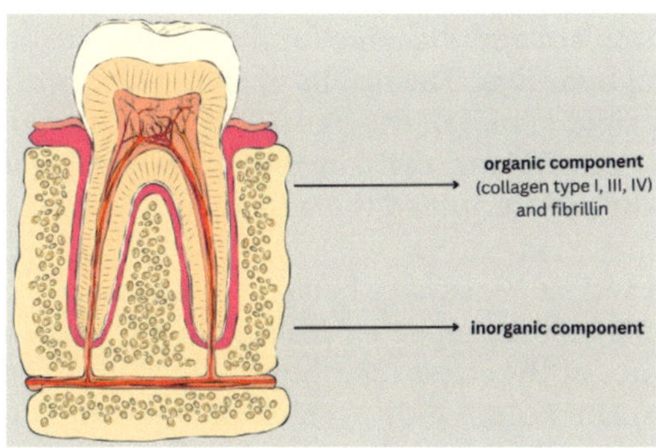

Figure 2.
Representation of the alveolar bone and its composition.

by hydroxyapatite [18]. The organic part offers flexibility to the entire structure, and the inorganic part is responsible for strength, summing their action during the presence of the tooth or implant in the alveolar bone (**Figure 2**). The entire architecture of the bone is responsible for the biological, chemical, and mechanical characteristics [19].

The bite forces exhibited by humans were reported to reach approximately 800 N in the molar, 600 N in the premolar, and 500 N in the canine region [20]. The mechanical forces and biological mechanisms are essential factors in order to induce and maintain the osteointegration process [21]. There are two different areas of the bone: the compact bone/cortical bone and the trabecular bone [22]. There are mechanical and biological differences between these areas, exhibiting different stiffness, creep and fatigue moduli, and tensile strength due to their different bone composition. Also, these properties can vary based on the anatomical site of the alveolar bone, patient's age, bone characteristics, and associated systemic conditions [23].

For an implant to be functional, the mechanical and biocompatibility properties are crucial for its good integration and functionality. The described mechanical properties of an implant are represented by their ability to resist the applied overdenture and added distributed forces, and these properties are divided into toughness, strength, stiffness, and ductility [24]. Related to stress resistance, there are several types that are in relation to the material and shape of the dental implant, the tensile, sheer, and compressive stress [25]. Also, the yield strength refers to the property of a material to resist stress without suffering from a plastic strain. The elastic modulus is represented by the rigidity of a material that has an implication in the strength and fatigue properties as well. The fatigue strength is a consequence of the composition and the suffered thermomechanical procedures. A higher fatigue strength has been associated with a long-term survival and functionality of the implants [26].

The implications of the design of the implant upon its mechanical properties and the osteointegration process are important aspects to be taken into consideration during the manufacturing stage.

The primary stability or the mechanical stability represents the result of the first interaction between the bone and the implant, without the implication of the biological process responsible for osteointegration [27]. During the osteointegration process, once the implant becomes biomechanically stable, the transition from the primary stability to the secondary stability is the key moment for prosthetic overload [28]. The further exhibited mechanical forces upon the implant need to correctly be distributed along the implant and the bone for the occurrence of bone resorption, due to progressive marginal bone loss. The results of an analysis outline two important aspects: When using a rigid material, the transfer of the resulted mechanical stress and deformation to the alveolar bone will be minimum, while the use of a material with a high elastic modulus determined the transfer of the stress to the surrounding alveolar bone [29].

Although titanium and its alloys have been used in dentistry, and especially implantology, their mechanical properties are not similar to the alveolar's bone, resulting in an imbalance of the stress distribution, leading eventually to bone resorption and secondary implant failure [30]. A solution would be the addition of other materials or manufacturing dental implants from other materials, in order to balance the mechanical forces and their distribution to the surrounding tissue.

2.2 Osteointegration of dental implants

During the placement of a dental implant, a series of changes occur in the soft and hard tissue, damaging and causing a local inflammatory response [31]. This response determines the further cellular interactions that will promote the local repair process. Particularly at this stage, the interaction between the mechanical forces and the biological local changes is the key for the osteointegration of the dental implant [21]. Studies have revealed that, in time, the interaction between the dental implant and the bone will form an effective biomechanical relationship with an important implication in the future stability and load forces once the implant is charged [32].

The individualized implant-prosthetic treatment should consider the interactions and changes that characterize the primary and secondary stability stages of an implant. While the primary stability is dependent on the surgical protocol, the shape, material, design, and bone characteristics, the secondary stability is based on the formation of new bone, a step that starts once the wound healing process begins. The understanding of these cellular and mechanical actions and their involvement in the osteointegration process is essential for the clinician to decide the proper time for loading the implant.

Aiming for efficient secondary stability, the new bone should form at the interface of the implant with the alveolar bone. Immediately after the surgical insertion of the

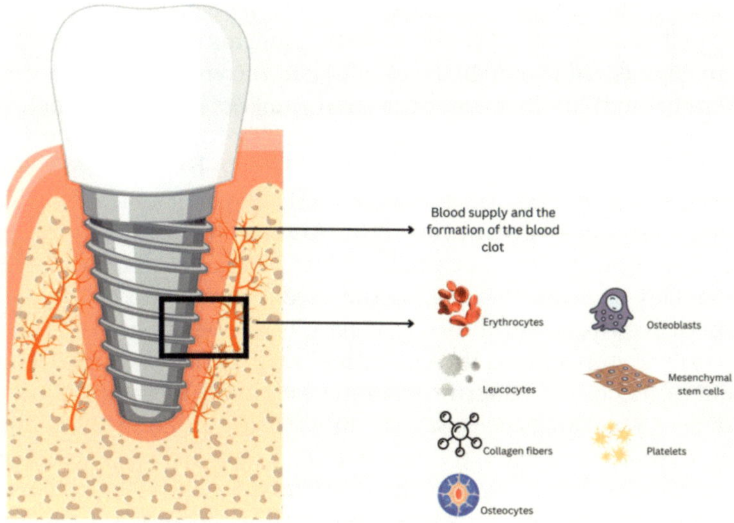

Figure 3.
Osteointegration of dental implants.

implant, the first step of the osteointegration starts by supplying the area with blood and eventually filling it with a blood clot [33]. The componence of the blood clot contributes to the local formation of granulation tissue due to the interaction of the mesenchymal stem cells and the newly formed vascularization [34] (**Figure 3**). The final stability of the dental implant is a result of the primary stability that decreases in the first 3 to 4 weeks and the secondary stability that increases by time [35].

Differences in the osteointegration process can occur due to the changes of the elastic modulus of the used materials. Studies have discussed that differences in the elastic modulus can have a negative effect upon the bone, determining peri-implant bone resorption [36]. Results have highlighted that the manufacture of dental implants with materials that exhibit a low elastic modulus has osteoconductive properties.

3. Composite dental implants

3.1 Polyetheretherketone (PEEK) dental implants

In implantology, the mechanical properties of the used dental materials are an important aspect to be taken into consideration. Currently, there are attempts in the development of new materials with modifications in their composition, in order to improve the existent inconveniences regarding the use of titanium and titanium-based alloys. Among the discussed mechanical changes are the fatigue and density properties that have direct repercussions upon the newly formed surrounding bone [37].

Among the developed materials are the polymeric ones, whose properties can be modified accordingly to their clinical purpose. Their mechanical behavior and structure can be designed to mimic the dental and bone structures, in order to achieve a desirable osteointegration process [38]. Polymers used for the manufacture of dental implants exhibited high fatigue and hardness levels, with an accurate deformation modulus that makes them an appealing approach for this restorative option [39].

PEEK is an engineered plastic that provides good strength, high biocompatibility, and good chemical stability in most of the environments [40]. Nevertheless, this type of polymer exhibits good mechanical properties and corrosion resistance, overcoming the reported disadvantages of titanium implants. Research studies outlined that PEEK implants compared to the titanium ones do not release particles and they do not determine an immune response from the host [40]. Another reported advantage was the fact that this type of polymer can be processed into different shapes and dimensions without influencing its properties, fitting the needs required for the dental implants. The high esthetic requirements of different areas of the dental arch can be fulfilled by using this type of implants, as their color is similar to the one of the alveolar bones and it does not influence the imagistic examination that uses magnetic resonance [41]. Nevertheless, regarding the elastic modulus that has an important impact upon the long-term stability of the dental implants, PEEK implants have a similar elastic modulus to the alveolar bone, limiting the stress transfer to the surrounding alveolar bone [42]. This type of polymer was approved by the Food and Drug Administration starting 1980 and has been successfully used also for orthopedic purposes [43].

Researchers have aimed to further improve the characteristics of this material by adding supplementary fillers such as glass and carbon fibers or hydroxyapatite in the PEEK matrix for maximizing the biomechanical properties [44–46]. The PEEK composites used for dental implants provided a high biocompatibility, having as well an important osteogenic activity and antimicrobial action [47]. By encapsulating the fillers in the matrix, their surface bioactive properties are still low, this being a further target for researchers [48]. By loading the PEEK composites with biomolecules, an improvement of the biochemical and biological characteristics was achieved, by developing a local environment that promotes cell growth and differentiation [49]. Liu et al. [50] in their study aimed to coat the surface of PEEK implants with titanium oxide (TiO_2) and activated by methacrylate hyaluronic acid in order to improve its properties. The results showed that the modified PEEK composites had higher hydrophilicity and promoted migration, adhesion, and proliferation of the human mesenchymal stem cells [50].

The osteointegration of the dental implants depends on the activity of the cellular growth factors. The fact that PEEK alone is an inert and hydrophobic material determines a low adherence of these growth factors that are the key for the new bone formation. In case of the PEEK coated with TiO_2, the adhesion of BMP-2 (bone morphogenic protein-2) was higher compared to PEEK implants alone, facilitating through a porous structure the adherence of BMP-2 to the surface of the implants [51]. In their study, Sun et al. [52] added and immobilized BMP-2 on the surface of PEEK implants, the results revealing a slow release of these proteins for the next 28 days. On the other hand, Guillot et al. [53], in the study they conducted, coated the PEEK implants with hyaluronic acid and loaded them with BMP-2. After their implantation in rabbits, they observed that, in case of the PEEK implants coated with BMP-2, the new bone formation was lower compared to the cases of using only PEEK implants. The explanation would be that the presence of local BMP-2 in high quantity determined the activation of osteoclasts and lower osteogenic activity. The conclusion was that the delivery of high levels of BMP-2 in the local environment should be avoided, having an initial antiosteogenic activity.

Studies reported that PEEK does not exhibit an antimicrobial property, offering an appealing environment for the plaque and bacterial adherence, with important consequences on the peri-implant tissue and long-term stability [54]. By adding

PDA coating with silver-ion, having a controlled release of the silver ions, the results showed a long-term antimicrobial activity [55]. Another approach to overcome this disadvantage of PEEK was the coating with sodium alginate hydrogel loaded with chlorogenic acid, exhibiting a significant antimicrobial activity upon Gram-positive and Gram-negative populations [56].

There have been intensive studies regarding the treatment of the surface of PEEK implants in order to achieve a bioactive product. One option presented by Khoury et al. [57] described the treatment of the surface using accelerated atom beams and reported an increase in the osteointegration of these implants without modifying their chemical structure. Another approach was presented by Poulsson et al. [58] by treating the surface of the implants with oxygen plasma for better osteointegration. A similar method was performed by Hassan et al. [59] that treated the surface with nitrogen plasma. Their results outlined a higher osteointegration rate compared to the one reported by using standard PEEK implants.

PEEK exhibits excellent mechanical and biological properties, and by adding filler materials, these properties can be improved in order to overcome the potential disadvantages that could influence the stability and osteointegration of these implants.

3.2 Bis-GMA and TEGDMA composite dental implants

Bis-GMA (bisphenol A-glycidyl methacrylate) and TEGDMA (triethylene glycol dimethacrylate) are categories of composites that have been recently introduced as potential materials for dental implants. Based on the properties they provide, although research has not focused on them related to this field, they can become a viable alternative to dental implants.

Resins are currently being used in dentistry for their high esthetic properties, decent strength, lower cost compared to ceramics, and capacity to form a bond with the structures of the teeth [60]. They have been classified as thermo-materials that can be reinforced with different fibers, such as glass fibers, in order for them to be successfully introduced in the implantology field.

Bis-GMA is a polymeric resin that has the property to penetrate easily into the printed samples, transforming into a strong material after polymerization. This characteristic makes them suitable for their integration as a matrix in the manufacture of dental implants [60].

Further *in vitro* studies aimed to evaluate the biological properties of this type of composite implant. A study aimed to assess the function of osteoblasts in relationship with HA-Bis-GMA. A culture of osteoblasts was analyzed after being in contact for several days with HA-Bis-GMA composites. The results revealed that the adherence of these cells to the composite surface was present, and their morphology did not suffer changes, highlighting the bioactive potential of this composite [61].

Chen et al. [62] reported that, by reinforcing the Bis-GMA composite with HA fibers, their properties can be improved by sintering methods, modifying their elastic modulus in order to be more similar to one of the alveolar bones.

The use of TEGDMA composite was assessed by combining it with Bis-GMA and bioactive glasses for the manufacture of dental implants in order to use two thermosets based on light-induced copolymerization. Abdulmajeed et al. [63] in their study aimed to evaluate the local response of the fibroblasts in relationship with these types of implants. The results reveal a higher adhesion of the fibroblasts on the surface of the implants manufactured from the combination of TEGDMA, Bis-GMA, and bioactive glasses.

3.3 Chitosan

Chitosan is a natural polymer, characterized by good biocompatibility, being biodegradable, and having the capacity to penetrate solid structures. In order to fulfill its purposes in the dentistry field, it is often associated with composites based on calcium phosphate, being reported an increase in the biomechanical properties, without interfering with the activity of the osteoblasts [64]. An *in vitro* study that focused on the use of hydroxyapatite and chitosan has reported an important exhibited osteoconductive action by promoting neovascularization as well [65].

One of the main advantages of this natural composite is its chemical composition due to the presence of hydrogen bonds that provide an increased resistance to heat [66]. This property is important when chitosan is combined with poly methylmethacrylate, needing a lower curing temperature [66]. Also, as studies observed, in time, the porous structure increases in dimension, outlining the biodegradable characteristic. The adherence of osteoblasts was also observed when coating the titanium implants with chitosan, suggesting the implication of coating in the osteointegration process of the standard used dental implants [64]. These properties provide an important perspective for the use of this type of material for the manufacture of dental implants.

4. Conclusions

Composite dental implants represent a viable option for the prosthetic rehabilitation of edentulous patients. Being described as biocompatible, osteoconductive, and with similar mechanical properties similar to the alveolar bone, composite dental implants represent a progress in the implantology field, overcoming the reported disadvantages of the standard titanium dental implants.

Conflict of interest

The authors declare no conflict of interest.

Author details

Alexandra Roi, Ciprian Roi*, Codruța Victoria Țigmeanu and Mircea Riviș
"Victor Babeș" University of Medicine and Pharmacy, Timișoara, Romania

*Address all correspondence to: ciprian.roi@umft.ro

References

[1] Albrektsson T, Branemark PI, Hansson HA, Lindstrom J. Osseointegrated titanium implants. Requirements for ensuring a long-lasting, direct bone-to-implant anchorage in man. Acta Orthopaedica Scandinavica. 1981;**52**:155-170

[2] Adell R, Hansson BO, Branemark PI, Breine U. Intra-osseous anchorage of dental prostheses. II. Review of clinical approaches. Scandinavian Journal of Plastic and Reconstructive Surgery. 1970;**4**:19-34

[3] Albrektsson T, Wennerberg A. The impact of oral implants – Past and future, 1966-2042. Journal of the Canadian Dental Association. 2005;**71**:327-327d

[4] Branemark PI, Adell R, Breine U, Hansson BO, Lindstrom J, Ohlsson A. Intra-osseous anchorage of dental prostheses. I. Experimental studies. Scandinavian Journal of Plastic and Reconstructive Surgery. 1969;**3**:81-100

[5] Branemark PI, Hansson BO, Adell R, Breine U, Lindstrom J, Hallen O. Osseointegrated implants in the treatment of the edentulous jaw. Experience from a 10-year period. Scandinavian Journal of Plastic and Reconstructive Surgery. Supplementum. 1977;**16**:1-132

[6] Schroeder A, Stich H, Straumann F, Sutter F. The accumulation of osteocementum around a dental implant under physical loading. SSO Schweiz Monatsschr Zahnheilkd. 1978;**88**:1051-1058

[7] Schulte W, Heimke G. The tubinger immediate implant. Die Quintessenz. 1976;**27**:17-23

[8] Schwitalla A, Müller WD. PEEK dental implants: A review of the literature. The Journal of Oral Implantology. 2013;**39**:743-749

[9] Bassir SH, El Kholy K, Chen CY, Lee KH, Intini G. Outcome of early dental implant placement versus other dental implant placement protocols: A systematic review and meta-analysis. Journal of Periodontology. 2019;**90**:493e506. DOI: 10.1002/JPER.18-0338

[10] Alghamdi HS, Jansen JA. The development and future of dental implants. Dental Materials Journal. 2020;**19**:167-e172. DOI: 10.4012/dmj.2019-140

[11] Li J, Jansen JA, Walboomers XF, van den Beucken JJ. Mechanical aspects of dental implants and osseointegration: A narrative review. Journal of the Mechanical Behavior of Biomedical Materials. 2020;**103**:103574

[12] Mouhyi J, Dohan Ehrenfest DM, Albrektsson T. The peri-implantitis: Implant surfaces, microstructure, and physicochemical aspects. Clinical Implant Dentistry and Related Research. 2012;**14**:170-183

[13] Schalock PC, Menné T, Johansen JD, et al. Hypersensitivity reactions to metallic implants diagnostic algorithm and suggested patch test series for clinical use. Contact Dermatitis. 2012;**66**:4-19

[14] Goutam M, Giriyapura C, Mishra SK, Gupta S. Titanium allergy: A literature review. Indian Journal of Dermatology. 2014;**59**:630

[15] Lee WT, Koak JY, Lim YJ, Kim SK, Kwon HB, Kim MJ. Stress shielding and

fatigue limits of poly-ether-ether-ketone dental implants. Journal of Biomedical Materials Research. Part B, Applied Biomaterials. 2012;**100**:1044-1052

[16] Le Gue Hennec L, Soueidan A, Layrolle P, Amouriq Y. Surface treatments of titanium dental implants for rapid osseointegration. Dental Materials. 2007;**2007**(23):844-854

[17] Annunziata M, Guida L. The effect of titanium surface modifications on dental implant osseointegration. Biomaterials for Oral and Craniomaxillofacial Applications. 2015;**17**:62-77

[18] Currey JD. The structure and mechanics of bone. Journal of Materials Science. 2012;**47**:41-54

[19] Wegst UGK, Bai H, Saiz E, Tomsia AP, Ritchie RO. Bioinspired structural materials. Nature Materials. 2015;**14**:23-36

[20] Brunski JB, Puleo DA, Nanci A. Biomaterials and biomechanics of oral and maxillofacial implants: Current status and future developments. The International Journal of Oral & Maxillofacial Implants. 2000;**15**:15-46

[21] Raghavendra S, Wood MC, Taylor TD. Early wound healing around endosseous implants: A review of the literature. The International Journal of Oral & Maxillofacial Implants. 2005;**20**:425-431

[22] Wu SL, Liu XM, Yeung KWK, Liu CS, Yang XJ. Biomimetic porous scaffolds for bone tissue engineering. Materials Science &Engineering R. 2014;**80**:1-36

[23] Winter W, Krafft T, Steinmann P, Karl M. Quality of alveolar bone - structure- dependent material properties and design of a novel measurement technique. Journal of the Mechanical Behavior of Biomedical Materials. 2011;**4**:541-548

[24] Ferraris S, Bobbio A, Miola M, Spriano S. Micro- and nano-textured, hydrophilic and bioactive titanium dental implants. Surface and Coating Technology. 2015;**2015, 276**:374383

[25] Anusavice KJ, Shen C, Rawls HR. Phillips' Science of Dental Materials. St.Louis, Misouri, US: Elsevier Health Sciences; 2012

[26] Abdel-Hady Gepreel M, Niinomi M. Biocompatibility of Ti-alloys for long-term implantation. Journal of the Mechanical Behavior of Biomedical Materials. 2013;**20Ș**:407-415

[27] Norton M. Primary stability versus viable constraint-a need to redefine. The International Journal of Oral & Maxillofacial Implants. 2013;**28**:19-21

[28] Gomes JB, Campos FE, Marin C, Teixeira HS, Bonfante EA, Suzuki M, et al. Implant biomechanical stability variation at early implantation times *in vivo*: An experimental study in dogs. The International Journal of Oral & Maxillofacial Implants. 2013;**2013**(28):E128-E134

[29] Perez-Pevida E, Brizuela-Velasco A, Chavarri-Prado D, Jimenez-Garrudo A, Sanchez-Lasheras F, Solaberrieta-Mendez E, et al. Biomechanical consequences of the elastic properties of dental implant alloys on the supporting bone: Finite element analysis. BioMed Research International. 2016;**2016**:1850401

[30] Gibson LJ, Ashby MF, Harley BA. Cellular Materials in Nature and Medicine. Cambridge, New York: Cambridge University Press; 2010

[31] Pellegrini G, Francetti L, Barbaro B, Del Fabbro M. Novel surfaces

and osseointegration in implant dentistry. Journal of Investigative and Clinical Dentistry. 2018;**9**:e12349

[32] Halldin A, Jimbo R, Johansson CB, Wennerberg A, Jacobsson M, Albrektsson T, et al. Implant stability and bone remodeling after 3 and 13 days of implantation with an initial static strain. Clinical Implant Dentistry and Related Research. 2014;**16**:383-393

[33] Salvi GE, Bosshardt DD, Lang NP, Abrahamsson I, Berglundh T, Lindhe J, et al. Temporal sequence of hard and soft tissue healing around titanium dental implants. Periodontology. 2000;**2015**(68):135-152

[34] Suzuki M, Calasans-Maia MD, Mann C, Granato R, Gil JN, Granjeiro JM, et al. Effect of surface modifications on early bone healing around plateau root form implants: An experimental study in rabbits. Journal of Oral and Maxillofacial Surgery. 2010;**2010**(68):1631-1638

[35] Bosshardt DD, Chappuis V, Buser D. Osseointegration of titanium, titanium alloy and zirconia dental implants: Current knowledge and open questions. Periodontology 2000. 2017, 2017;**73**:22-40

[36] Han X, Liu HC, Wang DS, Li SJ, Yang R, Tao XJ, et al. In vitro biological effects of Ti2448 alloy modified by micro-arc oxidation and alkali heatment. Journal of Materials Science and Technology. 2011;**27**:317-324

[37] Oladapo BI, Zahedi SA, Ismail SO, Omigbodun FT. 3D printing of PEEK and its composite to increase biointerfaces as a biomedical material- a review. Colloids and Surfaces. B, Biointerfaces. 2012;**203**:111726

[38] Oladapo BI, Zahedi SA, Adeoye AOM. 3D printing of bone scaffolds with hybrid biomaterials. Composites Part B: Engineering. 2019;**158**:428-436

[39] Oladapo BI, Obisesan OB, Oluwole B, Adebiyi VA, Usman H, Khan A. Mechanical characterisation of a polymeric scaffold for bone implant. Journal of Materials Science. 2020;**55**:9057-9069

[40] Kurtz SM, Devine JN. PEEK biomaterials in trauma, orthopedic, and spinal implants. Biomaterials. 2007;**28**:4845-4869

[41] Ma ZY, Zhao XY, Zhao J, Zhao ZI, Wang QH, Zhang CX. Biologically modified polyether ether ketone as dental implant material. Frontiers in Bioengineering and Biotechnology. 2020;**8**:620537

[42] Carpenter RD, Klosterhoff BS, Torstrick FB, Foley KT, Burkus JK, D. Lee CS, Gall K, Guldberg RE, Safranski DL. Effect of porous orthopaedic implant material and structure on load sharing with simulated bone ingrowth: A finite element analysis comparing titanium and PEEK. Journal of the Mechanical Behavior of Biomedical Materials. 2018;**80**:68-76

[43] He M, Huang Y, Xu H, Feng G, Liu L, Li Y, et al. Modification of polyetheretherketone implants: From enhancing bone integration to enabling multi-modal therapeutics. Acta Biomaterialia. 2021;**129**:18-32

[44] Zheng JB, Zhao HY, Ouyang ZC, Zhou XY, Kang JF, Yang CC, et al. Additively-manufactured PEEK/HA porous scaffolds with excellent osteogenesis for bone tissue repairing. Composites Part B: Engineering. 2022;**232**:109508

[45] Li Y, Wang DL, Qin W, Jia H, Wu Y, Ma J, et al. Mechanical properties,

hemocompatibility, cytotoxicity and systemic toxicity of carbon fibers/poly (ether-ether-ketone) composites with different fiber lengths as orthopedic implants. Journal of Biomaterials Science, Polymer Edition. 2019;**30**:1709-1724

[46] Lee WT, Koak JY, Lim YJ, Kim SK, Kwon HB, Kim MJ. Stress shielding and fatigue limits of poly-ether-ether-ketone dental implants. Journal of Biomedical Materials Research Part B-Applied Biomaterials. 2012;**100b**:1044-1052

[47] Wang LX, He S, Wu XM, Liang SS, Mu ZL, Wei J, et al. Polyetheretherketone/nano-fluorohydroxyapatite composite with antimicrobial activity and osseointegration properties. Biomaterials. 2014;**35**:6758-6775

[48] Cai GQ, Wang H, Jung YK, Xu ZY, Zhang JH, He JY, et al. Hierarchically porous surface of PEEK/nMCS composite created by femtosecond laser and incorporation of resveratrol exhibiting antibacterial performances and osteogenic activity *in vitro*. Composites Part B: Engineering. 2020;**186**:107802

[49] Zhang DY, Xu XY, Long XL, Cheng K, Li JS. Advances in biomolecule inspired polymeric material decorated interfaces for biological applications. Biomaterials Science. 2019;7:3984-3999

[50] Liu SD, Zhu YT, Gao HN, Ge P, Ren KL, Gao JW, et al. One-step fabrication of functionalized poly(etheretherketone) surfaces with enhanced biocompatibility and osteogenic activity. Materials Science & Engineering C-Materials for Biological Applications. 2018;**88**:70-78

[51] Han CM, Jang TS, Kim HE, Koh YH. Creation of nanoporous TiO_2 surface onto polyetheretherketone for effective immobilization and delivery of bone morphogenetic protein. Journal of Biomedical Materials Research. 2014;**102**:793-800

[52] Sun ZJ, Ouyang LP, Ma XH, Qiao YQ, Liu XY. Controllable and durable release of BMP-2-loaded 3D porous sulfonated polyetheretherketone (PEEK) for osteogenic activity enhancement. Colloids and Surfaces B: Biointerfaces. 2018;**171**:668-674

[53] Guillot R, Pignot-Paintrand I, Lavaud J, Decambron A, Bourgeois EE, Josserand V, et al. Assessment of a polyelectrolyte multilayer film coating loaded with BMP-2 on titanium and PEEK implants in the rabbit femoral condyle. Acta Biomaterialia. 2016;**36**:310-322

[54] D'Ercole S, Cellini L, Pilato S, Di Lodovico S, Iezzi G, Piattelli A, et al. Material characterization and *Streptococcus oralis* adhesion on polyetheretherketone (PEEK) and titanium surfaces used in implantology. Journal of Materials Science: Materials in Medicine. 2020;**31**:84

[55] Yu Y, Sun YM, Zhou X, Mao YR, Liu YX, Ye L, et al. Ag and peptide co-decorate polyetheretherketone to enhance antibacterial property and osteogenic differentiation, colloids surf. B-Biointerfaces. 2021;**198**:111492

[56] He X, Deng Y, Yu Y, Lyu H, Liao L. Drug-loaded/grafted peptide-modified porous PEEK to promote bone tissue repair and eliminate bacteria. Colloids and Surfaces. B, Biointerfaces. 2019;**181**:767-777

[57] Khoury J, Maxwell M, Cherian RE, Bachand J, Kurz AC, Walsh M, et al. Enhanced bioactivity and osseointegration of PEEK with accelerated neutral atom beam technology. Journal of Biomedical

Materials Research. Part B, Applied Biomaterials. 2015;**105**:531-543

[58] Poulsson AHC, Eglin D, Zeiter S, Camenisch K, Sprecher C, Agarwal Y, et al. Osseointegration of machined, injection moulded and oxygen plasma modified PEEK implants in a sheep model. Biomaterials. 2013;**35**:3717-3728

[59] Hassan AH, Al-Judy HJ, Fatalla AA. Biomechanical effect of nitrogen plasma treatment of polyetheretherketone dental implant in comparison to commercially pure titanium. Journal of Research in Medical and Dental Science. 2018;**6**:367-377

[60] Hosseinalipour M, Javadpour J, Rezaie H. Investigation of mechanical properties of experimental bis-GMA/TEGDMA dental composite resins containing various mass fractions of silica nanoparticles. Journal of Prosthodontics. 2010;**19**:112-117

[61] Suwanprateeb J, Sanngam R, Suwanpreuk W. Fabrication of bioactive hydroxyapatite/bis-GMA based composite via three dimensional printing. Journal of Materials Science. Materials in Medicine. 2008;**19**:2637-2645

[62] Chen L, Yu Q, Wang Y, Li H. BisGMA/TEGDMA dental composite containing high aspect-ratio hydroxyapatite nanofibers. Dental Materials. 2011;**27**:1187-1195

[63] Abdulmajeed AA, Kokkari AK, Käpylä J, Massera J, Hupa L, Vallittu PK, et al. In vitro blood and fibroblast responses to BisGMA–TEGDMA/bioactive glass composite implants. Journal of Materials Science: Materials in Medicine. 2014;**25**:151-162

[64] Di Martino A, Sittinger M, Risbud MV. Chitosan: A versatile biopolymer for orthopaedic tissue-engineering. Biomaterials. 2005;**26**:5983-5990

[65] Buranapanitkit B, Srinilta V, Ingviga N, Oungbho K, Geater A, Ovatlarnporn C. The efficacy of a hydroxyapatite composite as a biogradable antibiotic delivery system. Clinical Orthopaedics and Related Research. 2004;**424**:244-252

[66] Kim SB, Kim YJ, Yoon TL, Park SA, Cho IH, Kim EJ, et al. The characteristics of a hydroxyapatite–chitosan–PMMA bone cement. Biomaterials. 2004;**26**:5715-5723